Technology in Early Intervention

Infants & Young Children Series

Edited by

James A. Blackman, MD, MPH
Professor of Pediatrics
Director of Research
Kluge Children's Rehabilitation Center and Research Institute
Department of Pediatrics
University of Virginia
Charlottesville, Virginia

AN ASPEN PUBLICATION®
Aspen Publishers, Inc.
Gaithersburg, Maryland
1995

Library of Congress Cataloging-in-Publication Data

Technology in early intervention/
edited by James A. Blackman.
p. cm.
Consists of reprints of articles from Infants and young children.
Includes bibliographical references and index.
ISBN 0-8342-0649-8
1. Handicapped children—Rehabilitation—Technological innovations.
2. Rehabilitation technology.
3. Infants—Rehabilitation—Technological innovations.
I. Blackman, James A. II. Infants and young children.
[DNLM: 1. Rehabilitation—in infancy & childhood—collected works.
2. Rehabilitation—methods—collected works.
3. Technology—collected works.
4. Child Development—collected works.
WS 368 T255 1995]
RJ138.T43 1995
618.92—dc20
DNLM/DLC
for Library of Congress
94-39482
CIP

Editorial Services: Jane Colilla

Library of Congress Catalog Card Number: 94-39482
ISBN: 0-8342-0649-8
Series ISBN: 0-8342-0652-8

Printed in the United States of America

2 3 4 5

Table of Contents

Preface

Who has not been frustrated in trying to program the VCR only to find that the exciting conclusion to a movie was prematurely cut off? Or when the "save" key stroke on the word-processing program deletes a literary masterpiece? Or by struggling through the multiple choices of a voice mail system to talk with a humanoid?

Technology is here and it is wonderful, but sometimes it is exasperating, confounding, and downright inconvenient. Some people are technology junkies. They jump right in with the latest innovations before others are even aware of them. They have the latest upgrades, the quirkiest screen savers, and, of course, an internal double-speed CD player in the computer. They are the leaders; and, just as soon as the rest of us think we have caught up, they have moved on to another level.

Then there are the resistors. They claim ineptitude, visual-perceptual-motor weakness, or left-brain dominance, but the real problem is fear. Like former smokers who discover clean air, converts to technology wonder how they coped without it. Recidivism is commonplace, however. The resistors are completely content with the speed of a 486 processing chip. Forget multimedia add-ons.

Technology for technology's sake is a waste of time and financial resources. How many video cameras lie unused, perhaps unpacked, in early-intervention program storage closets? They may have been purchased because there was some left over money and someone thought their mere presence would update the program. Or they may be used indiscriminately with accumulation of boxes of uncatalogued, unedited tapes of the children. As part of a teaching program, visual records of children in therapy can be invaluable to parents, other family members, or to students. However, specific objectives must guide the use of technology for it to be of maximal value.

Technology is now available to assist in many of our activities: research, continuing education, case documentation, and developmental therapies. In some cases the technology may not be a gadget but a new technique or an innovative use of an old method.

The authors of the articles in this volume challenge us to consider some new approaches. The children and families we serve may benefit from technology if we first determine what it is they or we should hope to gain from it. Some children may be dependent on technology. Here the challenge is to incorporate it into the child's developmental plan or circumvent its limiting aspects. Through understanding we can make the best use of technology without becoming it slaves.

James A. Blackman, MD, MPH
Editor

High tech tots: Technology for mobility, manipulation, communication, and learning in early childhood

Charlene Butler, EdD
Special Educator
Seattle Public Schools
Child Development Mobility Consultant
Rehabilitation Department
Children's Hospital and Medical Center
Seattle, Washington

ARE VERY YOUNG children, even infants, really using technology successfully? What can these youngsters do with it? What is the justification for using advanced technology at this age? How can parents, teachers, and clinicians obtain information and learn how to make technology available to the young? This article answers these questions; raises some issues about the population from birth to 3 years using sophisticated technology; and suggests future applications.

WHY DO IT?

There is a growing realization that physical and psychologic development are interrelated and that early experiences influence subsequent behavior.[1] When development along any line is restricted, delayed, or distorted, other lines of development are adversely affected as well. Motor skills that develop rapidly during the first three years of life become the primary vehicle for learning and socialization. They foster a sense of competence and independence. Through their motor interactions, infants and toddlers learn about things and people in their world and also discover they can cause things to happen. They become active initiators and participants rather than passive recipients of experience.

Because most early handicapping conditions have a considerable motor component, disabled infants may lack the necessary movements to engage and act on their environment; thus, learning opportunities are hindered. Equally important, disabled infants' inability to influence their environment, that is, to affect or alter it through their own actions, leads to a condition of learned helplessness in which children give up trying to control their own world.[2] Repeated failure in exploring and mastering situations leads to a self-perception of incompetence and a passive resignation that extinguishes further attempts.[3] A sense of helplessness (or a sense of incompetence) is well established by 4 years of age.[4,5]

With the assistance of technology, disabled children can experience more success in directly controlling their environment, thereby reducing or avoiding secondary social-emotional and intellectual handicaps. The hope is that technology can take the handicap out of disabilities.

Inf Young Children 1988; 1(2): 66–73

WHAT CAN TECHNOLOGY DO?

Increasingly, opportunities for using technology are becoming available to the population from birth to age 3. Computer applications, powered mobility, myoelectric prostheses, and augmentative communication devices have been successfully demonstrated in research settings. Infants as young as 3 months have interacted with computers, 18-month-old children have driven powered mobility devices and used myoelectric hands, and 2-year-old children have talked via speech synthesizers. For severely physically disabled children, early intervention is focusing on teaching switch use and scanning techniques on which they may always have to rely for control of mobility, communication, independent learning, and environmental interaction. Competent school-entry users of these technologies may be able to achieve success in mainstream education.

MOBILITY

Clinical experience and research projects have established that powered mobility devices offer children at least as young as 17 months a safe and efficient method of independent locomotion.[6–8] The focus has been on the youngest age at which children can learn to use powered mobility, the manner in which they learn, and how it changes their behavior. There have been two primary concerns about powered aids for children: (1) the potential effect on ambulation and (2) safety.

Studies involving disabled 2 1/2- to 5-year-old children who were given specially designed electric carts focused on the risks, the children's psychosocial development, the level of supervision required, the development of and necessary level of driving skill, and the use they made of the devices.[9,10] No negative effects on motor development were noted. On the contrary, improved head control, trunk stability, and arm-hand function, increased motivation for physical training, and more self-confidence in movement activities were reported by parents and therapists. The few minor accidents included such things as banging into a tree while running away from parents or tilting over while making a too sharp turn in competition with friends on tricycles. Most children were skillful drivers well before a three-month, obstacle-course driving test. The carts were used most frequently for outside play, visits, and community activities. Increased independence in play and a decreased amount of physical assistance and supervision from parents were among the positive effects on psychosocial development.

Competent driving of motorized wheelchairs was reported for younger children (24 to 39 months).[11,12] They passed driving tests in an average of 16 days, which was the time taken by the youngest participant at 24 months. The driving test involved demonstration of driving in narrow corridors, turning, and maneuvering around people and objects. Since those reports, the youngest successful driver in the project has been 18 months of age. She, too, learned within three weeks and drove skillfully and safely. There were no worrisome accidents, and positive effects regarding motor behavior, social interactions, and emotional maturity were cited from parental reports.

One author,[13] studying six of the above children, focused on the effect of powered mobility on the frequency of self-initiated exploration of space, interaction with objects, and communication with caregivers. Three children showed increases in all three behaviors; one increased in communication and exploration; and two increased in spatial exploration only. The decreased communication for the last two children was regarded as positive, however, because they had been quite verbal and demanding. Independence through locomotion may have reduced their need for control through speech.

Devices designed to meet the needs of young children are becoming commercially available. The Turbo (Everaids Ltd, Cambridge, England), for example, is intended for children from 12 months of age and has such features as a "growing" seat and standing frame, variable height control, and ability to climb and descend curbs and to negotiate uneven terrain for outside play.[14]

The age at which devices are being prescribed is dropping at medical centers experimenting with technology for youngsters. Several recommend powered devices for children before age 3 and, in some cases, by 18 months. Most often, these are children with musculoskeletal disabilities, such as arthrogryposis and the dystrophies. Powered mobility has been tried with a few children as young as 11 and 12 months without success. Children who are too disabled to use a joystick can also learn, but the task is more complex and takes longer at any age.

MYOELECTRIC HANDS

At 18 months, children with congenital limb defects have demonstrated fluent use of small powered hands with only brief practice.[15,16] An electric motor, housed in the wrist and arm portion of the prosthesis, is activated by flexing the residual arm muscles. To use a myoelectric system, children are fit at 6 months with conventional prosthetic replacements for hands such as hooks. The conventional terminal device is progressively weighted in preparation for the heavier myoelectric hands. Current practice is to make the change to the myoelectric system at 18 months. There is no question that myoelectric hands are technically feasible for youngsters, but there is debate as to cost-effectiveness. The major issues are expense and practical value. Myoelectric hands are expensive in terms of original and replacement costs as the child grows. A service system must exist for maintenance and repair. Though more cosmetic and less cumbersome, it has not been established whether they are more functional (ie, whether they allow the child to do more activities faster or more efficiently than conventional prostheses). This option, therefore, is being pursued primarily in countries (eg, Sweden and Canada) with a social welfare system that purchases and maintains expensive technology.

MICROCOMPUTERS AND DEDICATED COMMUNICATION DEVICES

Considerable overlap exists between skills necessary for functional use of microcomputers dedicated to communication and microcomputers for independent learning. The same developmental prerequisites and access considerations apply to early-learning computer experiences of infants and toddlers and to augmentative communication.

Normal cognitive developmental literature suggests that infants have the requisite visual and cognitive abilities to begin using computers at about 8 months.[17] By this time, they can select objects from an array of picture options. By 15 months, infants can use computers as functional tools because they have sufficient planning ability even for use of a scanner for indicating a choice.

Computer access, however, is a problem for physically disabled youngsters who lack motor control to use a keyboard. If children can control one or two switches, access is possible through their action combined with a scanning strategy that highlights elements, rows, or columns of a matrix. The item selected could be a symbol or word to be communicated or it could be an instruction to an educational computer program. Once a reliable switch site or control point (eg, head, chin, knee) is identified, the child is trained in single- and dual-switch activation, scanning techniques, and encoding.

Sequential procedures and helpful software programs for teaching switch use in severely disabled children are being tested in clinical and research settings. One intervention design includes precomputer activities using a single switch to start and stop battery-operated toys and cause-effect software programs (eg, colors scroll across the screen) as an initial step.[18] After learning that switches produce interesting effects, the child progressively masters dual switches in order to initiate a scanning array and select a desired image as it is highlighted. Once this is achieved, increasingly complex scanning techniques are introduced, with the goal of speedy choice selection. A common hierarchy of scanning techniques begins with continuous scanning, moves through step or count scan, linear scan, and row-column scan, to directed scan, which can provide the most rapid choice making.

Attention is also being given to development of software for the teaching of higher-level cognitive skills beyond cause-effect relationships, which are necessary for independent use of both microcomputers and dedicated communication devices.[17–20] A gulf has existed between the few software programs to teach cause-effect and the relatively larger number of higher-function readiness programs that address the domains of visual discrimination, reading, and mathematics. Current research is focused on identification of interim skills and development of software to teach those skills. Skill hierarchy, other learner characteristics, equipment, and material features, as well as environmental factors that may affect success, are being explored.[17]

Augmentative communication

The youngest children using sophisticated vocal output systems for intentional speech are around 3 years old.[18] Sophisticated vocal output communication aids (VOCAs) have generally not been purchased for children below age 3. Clinicians cite a number of reasons. Usually children under age 3 do not produce complicated speech. Use of sophisticated systems requires cognitive understanding of how the communication software is organized and accessed. There must be sufficient motor control to make selections. Training in switch activation and scanning techniques with physically disabled children often takes a long time. High-quality, synthesized and new digitized speech hardware has been expensive and not portable enough for small children. The less expensive synthesized speech has been unacceptable to some clinicians because of their concerns about its intelligibility to youngsters and about children identifying with or imitating robot speech. Moreover, a training and service delivery system is lacking to provide for maintenance and for upgrades to more sophisticated communication software as language needs become more complex. Finally, the current therapy model, which features long-term, intermittent training, is inadequate. Over the short term, intensive training periods are needed for children to become skillful users of sophisticated technology.

Parents and clinicians in some areas, however, are routinely referring children from 15 to 18 months old for consideration of augmentative communication. For age-appropriate expressive language, children need early acquisition of the skills (ie, switch activation, scanning, encoding) necessary for use of VOCAs. Two-year-olds are using simple vocal output aids. Given the new developments in digitized speech technology, it is conceivable that inexpensive and simple VOCAs will be used increasingly, even with infants, for production of speech and language precursors like babbling. Guides for training expressive communication from the neonatal period, including early intervention with technology, are increasingly available.[21,22] Revision of Minspeak (Prentke Romich, Wooster, Ohio), powerful communication software designed for older children and adults, is also underway for children younger than 3. Experimentation with early introduction of the concepts on which it is based is said to show promise.

Learning with microcomputers

Research on utilization of microcomputers with young disabled children below age 3 is just beginning to emerge in the literature. Three types of applications have been reported. One has been valuable for direct training of sensorimotor skills.[23] In another, contingency awareness was stimulated in children who could not manipulate objects in their environment or play together and who displayed little interest in anything.[24] In both of these applications, the computer was also a powerful management tool. Its ability to quickly analyze large amounts of complex data allowed more precise shaping of behavior through immediate reinforcement of desired behavior. Even the nature of the reinforcement could be programmed for continual adjustment based on input as to the child's level of interest. In addition, the data on child behavior could help in determining needed changes in body positioning or switch placement. Finally, the microcomputer stimulated communication and socialization through cooperative use of early childhood software programs.[25]

The computer-based system for teaching gross motor skills to multiply disabled toddlers used an integrated combination of adaptive positioning equipment, individualized switches, battery-operated toys, and a microcomputer.[23] The microcomputer monitored and reinforced (1) sitting erect; (2) reaching, grasping, and pulling; and (3) trunk extension from kneeling. It also monitored teacher behavior (ie, physical assists). The monitoring data were used to modify training, increasing the precision with which these gross motor skills could be taught. Increased frequency and duration of the three target motor skills were demonstrated in generalized settings as well as in the training sessions.

Combined use of adaptive switches and microcomputers helped train contingency awareness or cause-effect relationships in children as young as 3 months who had mentally retarding conditions such as Down syndrome.[24] When children learn that they can cause things to happen, they become more interested and involved in their environment. Twenty-one children (3 to 6 months of age) learned to use a variety of input devices to activate microcomputer-driven objects such as toys and systematically varied their behavior to explore specific contingencies.

Microcomputer activities stimulated communication in children who did not talk because of psychologic barriers or because of severely limited experiences. Clinical work has demonstrated that computer activities stimulate speech in youngsters by providing novel, interesting experiences to talk about.[25] Exciting, interactive software, shared with another child or adult, provides an intent, a purpose, and relevant reinforcement for communication.

Use of computer technology is increasing rapidly despite current lack of appropriate software, hardware funding, and teacher training. Results of a survey of 52 directors of early childhood special education programs, enrolling a population from birth to 5 years, showed that more than half of their programs were using computers or had plans to do so.[26] Project ACTT (Activating Children Through Technology) reports increasing requests for teacher training workshops and outreach programs. At the Virginia Preschool Technical Assistance Centers, approximately 90% of over 300 requests for help in 1987 specified technology. This percentage was up from approximately 5% in previous years.

OBTAINING INFORMATION ABOUT TECHNOLOGY APPLICATIONS

Already a number of organizations are devoted to demonstrating the positive impact technology can have on the lives of children with disabilities. Most are listed in the *Resource Directory* published annually by Closing the Gap, Inc. Closing the Gap has workshops, consultations, an annual international conference, and a newspaper published six times a year. Closing the Gap offers, perhaps, the most up-to-date reports available on technology uses in special education and rehabilitation for children. Its *Resource Directory* is thorough and offers an easy-to-use guide to technology products and distributors, as well as organizations.

Descriptions of innovative or helpful uses of technology, products, and processes are available from ACTT, Handicapped Children's Early Education Project (HCEEP), and Innotek (see box). These projects provide excellent resources and offer technology assessment and application workshops. The Pennsylvania Special Education Assistive Device Center provides assistance, training, and short-term loans of technology devices through local school systems. Catalogs from companies that distribute technology-based products are informative. Rehabilitation departments of university-affiliated hospitals, such as Tufts, University of Tennessee, University of Washington, Stanford, and the Hugh McMillan Center (Toronto), are also in the forefront of technology development for disabled children and can provide information and direction to service providers.

Resources

1. ACTT (Activating Children Through Technology), Macomb Projects, 27 Horrabin Hall, Western Illinois University, Macomb, IL 61455.
2. HCEEP (Handicapped Children's Early Education Project), Technical Assistance Development System, North Carolina University, Chapel Hill, NC 27514.
3. Innotek, Division of National Lekotek Center, 2100 Ridge Ave., Evanston, IL 60201.
4. Pennsylvania Special Education Assistive Device Center, Elizabethtown Hospital and Rehabilitation Center, Elizabethtown, PA 17022.
5. Closing the Gap, P.O. Box 68, Henderson, MN 56044.
6. Preschool Technical Assistance Center, George Mason University, Fairfax, VA 22030.

REFERENCES

1. Rosenbloom L: Consequences of impaired movement: A hypothesis and review, in Hold KS (ed): *Movement and Child Development.* Philadelphia, Lippincott, 1975, pp 159–162.
2. Lewis M, Goldberg S: Perceptual-cognitive development in infancy: A generalized expectancy model as a function of the mother-infant interaction. *Merrill-Palmer Q* 1969;15:81–100.
3. Harter S: Effectance motivation revisited: Toward a developmental model. *Human Dev* 1978;21:34–64.
4. Safford PL, Arbitman DC: *Developmental Intervention with Young Physically Handicapped Children.* Springfield, Ill, Charles C Thomas, 1975.
5. Kohn M: Social competence, in *Symptoms and Underachievement in Childhood: A Longitudinal Perspective.* New York, Wiley, 1977.
6. Zazula JL, Foulds RA: Mobility device for a child with phocomelia. *Arch Phys Med Rehabil* 1983;64:137–139.
7. Rehabilitation Engineering Center: *Third Annual Report.* Palo Alto, Children's Hospital at Stanford, 1977.
8. Orthokenetics: *Pediatrics Rehabil Newsletter* 1985;4(January/February):2.
9. Paulsson K, Christoffersen M: Psychological aspects of technical aids: How does independent mobility affect the psychological and intellectual development of children with physical disabilities? *Proceedings of the Second Annual Conference on Rehabilitation Engineering.* Ottawa, Canada, 1984. Washington, DC, RESNA, 1984, pp 282–286.
10. Verburg G, Snell E, Pilkington M, et al: Effects of powered mobility on young handicapped children and their families. *Proceedings of the Second Annual Conference on Rehabilitation Engineering.* Ottawa, Canada, 1984. Washington, DC, RESNA, 1984, pp 172–173.
11. Butler C, Okamoto GA, McKay T: Powered mobility for very young disabled children. *Dev Med Child Neurol* 1983;25:472–474.
12. Butler C, Okamoto GA, McKay T: Motorized wheelchair driving by disabled children. *Arch PHM* 1984;65:95–97.
13. Butler C: Effects of powered mobility on self-initiated behaviors of very young children with locomotor disability. *Dev Med Child Neurol* 1986;28:325–332.
14. Jaffe KM, Butler C, Hayes RM, et al: An innovative motorized wheelchair for young disabled children. *J Assoc Child Pros-Ortho Clin* 1986;21:46–51.
15. Sorbye R: Myoelectric prosthetic fitting in young children. *Clin Orthop* 1980;148:34–40.
16. Scott RN, Dunfield VA, Richard PD, et al: Myoelectric control system for young children. *Inter-Clinic Infor Bull* 1983;19:4–5.
17. Porter L, Lahm L, Behrmann MM, et al: Designing picture based software for the cognitively young. *J Div Early Child* 1986;10:231–239.
18. Hutinger PL: Computers, communication, and young handicapped children: A winning combination. *Closing the Gap* April–May 1987:12.
19. Warren SF, Horn EM: Microcomputer applications in early childhood special education: Problems and possibilities. *Top Early Childhood Ed* 1987;7:72–83.
20. Behrmann MM, Lahm L: Babies and robots: Technology to assist learning of young multiply disabled children. *Rehabil Lit* 1984;45:194–201.

21. Burkhart LJ: *Using Computers and Speech Synthesis to Facilitate Communicative Interaction with Young and/or Severely Handicapped Children.* College Park, Md, (self-published), 1987.
22. Blackstone SW, Bruskin DM (eds): *Augmentative Communication: An Introduction.* Rockville, Md, ASHA, 1986.
23. Horn EM, Warren SF: Facilitating the acquisition of sensorimotor behavior with a microcomputer-mediated teaching system: An experimental analysis. *J Assoc Severe Handicap* 1987;12:205–215.
24. Brinker RP, Lewis M: Making the world work with microcomputers: A learning prosthesis for handicapped infants. *Except Child* 1982;49:163–170.
25. Hutinger PL: Computers and young handicapped children: More on communication. *Closing the Gap* June–July 1987:16,17,19,20.
26. Gold RR: Use of microcomputers in New York State early childhood special education programs. Paper presented at Annual Meeting of Eastern Educational Research Association, Virginia Beach, Va, Feb 7–9, 1985.

Technology intervention for very young children with disabilities

Michael M. Behrmann, EdD
Director
Center for Human Disabilities

Julie K. Jones, PhD
Coordinator
Severely Profoundly Handicapped
Technical Assistance Center

Mary L. Wilds, MAEd
Coordinator
Early Childhood Handicapped
Technical Assistance Center No. 3
George Mason University
Fairfax, Virginia

WHEN MOST persons think of the information age, brought on by the profusion of microcomputers and microprocessor-based technology, they generally do not consider applications for very young children, particularly children with handicaps. Although software and hardware for preschool children are no longer rare, development of technology applications for very young children and children with disabilities is limited. Recent federal legislation should do much to encourage continued development of computer technologies, software, and most importantly, innovative approaches to apply these technologies. On August 19, 1988, President Reagan signed Public Law 100-407, the Technology-Related Assistance for Individuals with Disabilities Act of 1988. This legislation is designed to assist states in designing technology-related assistance for all disabled individuals, including very young children. Additionally, the passage of Public Law 99-457 in 1986, the amendments to the Education of All Handicapped Children's Act of 1975, provides states with incentives to provide educational interventions to handicapped children from birth to two years of age as well as to provide funds for technology-related research and development in special education.

This article focuses on technology applications that can be used by children with disabilities from birth to three years of age, primarily those with more severe handicaps and sensory impairments. Many of the activities suggested in the article may also be useful with children who are at risk, have attention deficit disorders, or need to develop appropriate socialization skills. Two notes of caution should be taken by the reader. First, it is often difficult to determine whether a young child is cognitively intact. One cannot assume that a child with multiple handicaps is also retarded. The appropriate application of technology can assist professionals and families in learning about a child's capabilities. Another variable to consider here is whether the child is motivated by the activities provided. Some children are just disinterested or bored by the materials, not cognitively impaired. The second caution is that technology is not the answer to every child's problems. There are often significant frustrations associated with using technology with young handicapped children, and each child must be individually assessed to determine the potential benefits of technology. Also, many disabled children are able to learn in the same

Inf Young Children 1989; 1(4): 66–77

ways as nondisabled children. While technology interventions can provide some advantages to some children, it is important to allow children to learn in normal ways whenever possible.

TOOLS FOR LEARNING, RECREATION, AND LIVING

The advent of microprocessor technology has infiltrated virtually every component of society in the United States during the last ten years. Some would say it greatly facilitates daily living for nearly everyone. Others feel that it greatly complicates daily living. Whatever the case, it is now difficult to avoid the use of these technologies. For instance, automated banking tellers and telephones that signal incoming calls are but two examples of the daily use of microprocessors. Applications of technology even extend to very young children through the introduction of toys that talk or otherwise respond to children's actions. Microprocessor-based toys and other applications of technology developed specifically for individuals with disabilities are providing new tools for learning, recreation, and living for children with disabilities.[1]

As a tool for learning, technology can provide access to traditional academic and readiness activities such as learning to recognize letters or numbers. It can also provide a means for children with severe physical handicaps to learn independently by manipulating their environment. For instance, by turning battery-operated toys on and off using simple switches, children who are otherwise physically unable to actively participate in learning activities can now engage in appropriate learning activities consistent with the developmental learning stages noted by Piaget and others.[2]

New tools for recreation are also available using technology. Recreation implies the concept of play, which is a critical component of any curriculum for very young children. Single-switch controls allow young children to turn on a television and videocassette recorder, change channels, listen to music on a tape recorder, control battery-operated toys, and otherwise independently engage in play activities. Art and music are also made available. For instance, a child who is unable to hold a crayon can use a graphics software package to move a cursor and create a line drawing, or press a switch and fill in color in a paint-by-numbers drawing. A color graphics printer can then draw the picture and the child can take it home for display on the refrigerator.

As a tool for living, technology provides children with disabilities access to new means of interacting with people and environments. In addition to controlling electrical and battery-operated objects, augmentative communication devices now provide new ways of interacting with peers, parents, teachers, and others. Children unable to verbalize can now speak to others using improved voice synthesis, a range of symbol sets and systems, and unique ways of transmitting language efficiently.

TECHNOLOGY INTERVENTION

When investigating appropriate models of technology intervention with very young children, it is important to diverge from a traditional preschool educational model of intervention, which focuses on domains such as reading readiness and fine motor skills. With very young children with disabilities, technology should be viewed as a means to provide new methods of access to play, language, and socialization, the primary developing domains of young children.

There has not been a substantial amount of research on technology intervention with very young children. Brinker and Lewis[3] have used microcomputers to illustrate that handicapped infants (three to five months old) can learn cause and effect relationships using a switch. They used a contingency-intervention approach in which pressing a switch resulted in a microcomputer-controlled contingency. They determined that the microcomputer was able to foster a generalized expectancy by handicapped infants that the world was controllable, and they were able to lead infants to use specific behavioral movements to explore the contingencies available. Their intervention was based on the developmental range from primary circular reactions to simple means-ends behavior.[4]

Behrmann and Lahm[5,6] have conducted studies and written a number of papers related to using computers with infants and toddlers. These studies were designed to determine the functional skills necessary to interact with technology and to develop methods to teach infants and toddlers to use a microcomputer to select options (make choices) that resulted in activating electrical toys and devices in their environment. They were concerned with teaching the skills necessary for learning to use a scanning mechanism to make choices for a child unable to make a direct selection due to a physical handicap. These skills include the ability to survey the options, make a decision, know where the scanning pointer is located, visually track the scanner, and initiate an appropriate motor movement to activate the switch that would effect the selection. They concluded that technology can be used to teach very young children these skills. They also noted the importance of providing the child with opportunities to play, or experiment, with the results of their interactions with the technology. This early work showed that very young children could use computer technology. Therefore, the issue was raised of providing very young handicapped children with the opportunity to take an active role in learning through the use of technology.

The positive effects of early intervention are well documented in special education literature.[7] Providing children with technology-based opportunities to interact with their learning environment can teach children to be independent rather than dependent learners.

Porter et al[8] completed a literature review on software developed for cognitively impaired young children. They identified the critical factors and skills necessary to use computer software. Their review indicated that available software for this population falls into two categories: (1) that designed to teach cause and effect through the use of a microcomputer and (2) that which focuses on teaching content areas such as the labeling of pictures and objects. They also determined that this software tends to be picture based using color, movement, sound, and shape and often supplemented with voice synthesis. Their review suggests that computer software can (and should) be developed for very young handicapped children.

Other researchers[9–11] have been concerned with symbolic representation as it relates to use of augmentative communication devices. The presentation of choices for very young children obviously needs to involve some type of representation of referents (eg, real objects, photographs, pictures, line drawings, symbols). Of great concern, then, is how symbolic these representations can be when dealing with very young children. If they cannot associate the representations with their referents, they would obviously be hindered in using their communication devices. While many assume that the ability to recognize and interpret representations exists in some type of hierarchy,[9–11] research does not support this assumption.[9,11] Individualizing symbol selection will ensure the best match between child and representation.[9]

While there has been relatively little research conducted on technology intervention with very young children, the research that has been done has provided the rationale for a number of projects across the United States. Handicapped Children's Early Education Projects such as the Macoomb Project's Activating Children Through Technology (ACTT)[12] were supported by the Office of Special Education and Rehabilitative Services in the U.S. Department of Education. Public Law 99-457 has also had an effect on projects for very young children through incentives for programs for the birth to two-year population. For example, Virginia's Early Childhood Handicapped Technical Assistance Centers (TACs), particularly TAC No. 3 at George Mason University, have provided technical assistance in technology to programs serving handicapped infants and toddlers as well as the more traditional three to five year population. The Virginia State Department of Education has also responded to the demand for technology training and technical assistance for personnel serving preschool handicapped children by funding a statewide TAC Technology Coordinator to provide this assistance on a statewide basis.

Skills necessary for technology use

Many persons working with very young children with handicaps can see many potential benefits to using technology with these children. However, it is critically important to realize three things. First, there are not a tremendous number of technology applications available for this population (either software for computers or adaptive devices). Second, many skills are necessary for using this technology effectively, and most of these skills can be developed without access to expensive computers or technological devices. Third, current state-of-the-art technology does not provide adequate hardware and software to teach all of the necessary skills. While many of these skills are discussed in more detail in the articles mentioned previously, Wilds[13] summarizes the skills necessary for effective infant and preschool technology use as follows:

- Motor skills
  - range of motion
  - press and release
  - reliable and consistent motor movement
- Visual/perceptual skills
  - visual tracking and scanning
  - figure ground
  - form discrimination
- Cognitive/language skills
  - cause and effect
  - attention span (sustained or selective)
  - object permanence
  - means/ends causality
  - imitation
  - one-to-one correspondence
  - intentional behavior (desire to communicate)
  - symbolic representation (recognize pictures)
  - reliable yes/no response
  - receptive understanding of commands
  - making choices
- Social/emotional skills
  - initiating and terminating interactions
  - turn taking and waiting for turn
  - attending to an object or person
  - following one-step directions

While this list of skills may initially seem overwhelming, their training can be included in activities relatively easy to incorporate into infant and early preschool curricula using adapted toys and switches when other appropriate hardware and software are not available. These activities can then be expanded to augmentative communication devices and other assistive devices as well as to computer-based activities.

Integrating toys and switches into the curriculum

The importance of play for very young children cannot be overemphasized when developing a curriculum. Thus, the tools of teaching are often toys that are concrete and motivating to children. For children who are physically handicapped or are generally uninterested in manipulative toys, battery-operated toys that are adapted to work with single switches can be used. Goosens' and Crain[14,15] suggest that battery-operated toys reflecting a variety of sensory inputs should be used. This approach encourages the use of various sensory modalities by the children while at the same time providing enough variation to maintain motivation by avoiding boredom. Visual sensory input can be obtained with toys that have flashing or blinking lights. Auditory input can be through tape recordings, music, or other sounds. Tactile input is available with fans or vibrating toys. The toys should also have a variety of movement and sensory features. A bear banging a drum shows stationary repetitive movement combined with auditory input, and a police car or robot provides horizontal movement often combined with light and sound. Vertical movement can also be shown by a toy firefighter climbing a ladder. Toys such as these can be incorporated into interactive play and can illustrate and reinforce cognitive development and language.

Virtually any toy that is battery operated can be inexpensively adapted to be operated by a single switch. Battery interrupters, devices that are placed between the battery and on/off switch to conduct current through the adaptive switch, can be made[16] and connected to electronic switches. Switches can also be inexpensively made using components available at a local electronics store. If desirable, commercial switches as well as already adapted toys can be purchased for as little as $20 (see boxed material).

A variety of switches that can activate toys is also desirable, since children present a hierarchy of learning needs as well as having different physical requirements. At the lowest levels, the switch can be integrated into the device that is activated, thus establishing a cause and effect relationship. That is, the device makes sounds or vibrates when it is touched. At the next level, a toy is plugged into a separate switch, which activates the toy. This level requires that the child cognitively understands the cause and effect relationship as well as the relationship between the switch and a device not directly associated with the switch. At this level, activation of a toy can be tied to representational or symbolic play where communication skills can be a focus. Socialization activities can also be introduced at this level, having children take turns activating the toy and playing together or in parallel play. At the next level, two switches activating different toys can be introduced, providing opportunities to engage the child in selective discrimination or choice-making tasks. This can be made even more complex by introducing one switch that has two activators, such as a rocker switch.

When working with infants and toddlers with physical disabilities, access to a variety of switches is imperative. Finding an appropriate switch or switches that match the child's physical requisites is extremely important. The child must have a reliable motor movement that can consistently activate the toy. As the child becomes more capable, the more reliable motor movements available to activate

Sources for Toys/Switches and Computer Use with Infants and Preschoolers

ABLENET, Accessibility, Inc, 360 Hoover Street NE, Minneapolis, MN 55413, (612) 331-5958.

Adamlab, Wayne County Intermediate School District, 33500 Van Born Road, Wayne, MI 48184.

Adaptive Communication Systems, Inc (ACS), PO Box 12440, Pittsburgh, PA 15231, (412) 264-2288.

Colorado Easter Seal Society for Handicapped Children and Adults, Inc, 5755 West Alameda Avenue, Lakewood, CO 80226.

Communication Aids for Children & Adults, Crestwood Company, PO Box 04606, Milwaukee, WI 53204-0606, (312) 526-9876.

Don Johnston Developmental Equipment, PO Box 639, 1000 North Rand Road, Bldg 115, Wauconda, IL 60084, (312) 526-2682.

Dunamis, Inc, 2856 Buford Highway, Duluth, GA 30136.

Innocomp, 33195 Wagon Wheel Drive, Solon, OH 44139.

Kanor, Steven, PhD, 8 Main Street, Hastings-on-Hudson, NY 10706, (914) 478-0960.

Laureate Learning Systems, Inc, 100 East Spring Street, Winooski, VT 05404, (802) 655-4755.

Microcomputers Systems for the Handicapped: *Choice Maker.* 10418 Armstrong Street, Fairfax, VA 22030.

Phonetica One, Inc, 4089 Dover Drive, Colorado City, CO 81019.

Prentke Romich Company, 1022 Heyl Road, Wooster, OH 44691.

Schell, G: *How to Make Toys and Training Aids for Handicapped Children.* LTV Aerospace and Defense Company (LTVAD), PO Box 225907, Dallas, TX 75265.

Sunburst Communications, 39 Washington Avenue, Pleasantville, NY 10570.

TASH (Technical Aids and Systems for the Handicapped), Inc, 70 Gibson Drive, Unit #12, Markham, Ontario, Canada L3R 4C2, (416) 475-2212.

UCLA/LAUSD Microcomputer Software, 1000 Veterans Avenue, Rm. 23-10, Los Angeles, CA 90024.

Unicorn Engineering Co, 6201 Harwood Avenue, Oakland, CA 94618.

Xerox (Weekly Reader Family Software), 4343 Equity Drive, PO Box 16754, Dept. MS13, Columbus, OH 43216.

switches will provide a means of more efficiently interacting with his or her environment. Recent technology has provided a variety of mechanisms for these children to activate toys other than simply using a switch activated by pressing it with their hand. For example, children can use an eye-blink switch or a puff switch to activate a device. Pressure switches that require only a minimal amount of movement are now on the market. Voice activation of devices is also now possible. There are electronic toys on the market such as Fred the stuffed dog by Phonetica One Inc, a robotic toy that responds to vocalizations, or the Cabbage Patch Talking Kids that respond to sounds children make.[17] Pointing switches such as infrared devices and eye-gaze switches are also available, though their costs are generally much greater, and infants and toddlers generally do not have the cognitive skills to use such switches. These switch interfaces are often associated with more sophisticated devices, such as augmentative communication devices.

Augmentative communication and technology

A segment of the very young children addressed in this article requires a discussion of the issues related to augmentative communication and technology-enhanced language development. For these children, whose verbal communication is particularly difficult or physically not possible, technology with a purpose (ie, communication) provides substantial motivation to develop the skills necessary to interact with technology. Thus it is another important approach in integrating technology into the curriculum.

Advances in the use of technology for communication are now returning passively observing young children with physical disabilities to active participation in the communication process. Both dedicated augmentative communication devices and computers modified with peripherals can now open communication channels for these very young children. In addition and equally important, they provide ways for these children to receive communication training that is interactive in nature, allowing them to practice communication skills independently without relying on one-to-one interactions with practitioners.

Devices developed as dedicated augmentative communication devices are known as vocal output communication aids, or VOCAs. Several companies have developed devices appropriate for use with very young children. Prentke Romich Company, for example, has developed the Touch Talker, Light Talker, and IntroTalker. Adaptive Communication Systems markets the Alltalk and Speech PAC, while Adamlab markets the Wolf and Scan Wolf and Innocomp the Say-It-All. These devices come equipped with modifiable displays, programmable software, and synthetic speech. As a result, they allow for individualization of vocabulary and organization of content as well as for freedom of choice of display symbols (eg, objects, photographs, line drawings). These sophisticated systems can also grow as the communication abilities of the children expand.

Similarly, computers can be used to meet the communication needs of very young children with disabilities. Practitioners can add peripheral devices such as the Muppet Learning Keys by Sunburst, the Power Pad by Dunamis, and Unicorn Keyboard by Unicorn Engineering to enlarge, extend, and simplify the computer keyboard. They can add voice via an add-on synthesizer such as the Echo Voice synthesizer by Street Electronics. By using software such as the *Talking PowerPad* by Dave Schmitt of the Colorado Easter Seal's Computer Resource Center (public domain) or *Talking Unicorn Board* by Unicorn Engineering, they can create simple or sophisticated individualized communication programs for many children. Sometimes practitioners may prefer to begin a young child on a simple computerized communication program before moving the child to an augmentative device.

Matching device and child is a complicated process, requiring many of the skills discussed in the previous section to obtain success. Many factors must be considered. First, finding the best method for accessing the devices is critical. Frequently, the switch or activation device the child has been using to activate toys will transfer to his or her communication devices. Other times, providing a touch pad is desirable.

Second, the method of selecting an option for communication is important. If possible, direct selection of the option is the fastest and most preferred input choice. This simply involves selecting the desired item by touching one of the appropriate squares or display portions from an array of options on the device. If direct selection is not possible, several types of scanning techniques are available for those who are unable to select their communication choices directly. The Light Talker, for example, offers 23 different scanning techniques. Basically, scanning is a technique whereby a person, pointer, or moving light offers selections from which the child (the communicator) chooses. Linear, circular, and row-column are all scanning techniques. Practitioners need to be judicious in choosing a scanning method with very young children because what may ultimately be the best input method for communication may not be the one to begin working with. For example, item selection via multiswitch-directed scanning may need to be taught first through row-column scanning with a single switch. In some instances, scanning may need to be used before introducing a more sophisticated direct-selection method. For example, direct selection using an infrared light mounted on the head is generally not viable for very young children. Direct selection through this more sophisticated device can then be introduced when the child is ready.

A third factor to consider in device selection is the positioning needed for the child to interact with the communication device. If the device can be used only while seated in a chair and the child spends more time outside a chair, that device may not be the best choice.

How well a system will be able to change to meet communicative needs is a fourth concern when looking at devices for very young children. Some systems provide for multiple (and often complex) input for efficient communication, which becomes increasingly important as communicative abilities increase. Other systems require shifting overlays frequently in order to access sufficient vocabulary as the communicative abilities of the children expand. How quickly the children can access what they want to say is especially important with very young children, who are not noted for long attention spans and patience.

A fifth and final important consideration, especially from the parents' perspective, involves the cost and benefits of devices. The range of costs is quite broad. The Wolf and Scan-Wolf, for example, cost under $350, while the Light Talker with needed switches and mounting can cost over $4,000. On the other hand, the Light Talker, which can be interfaced to a computer, would probably be the only device ever needed, while a less expensive device probably will need to be upgraded. The roles that the device will play in the total communication and learning opportunities for the child are also a part of determining cost *v* benefits.

Simply supplying young children with a way of communicating is not sufficient to provide children with the learning opportunities that non-communicatively impaired children have. What technology has done is provide a means of communicating or, for many, a means of communicating more easily. It does not, however, automatically transform them into active communicators. Training is necessary for them to take advantage of this communication technology. As with the devices and programs, such training must be individualized and matched to each child. In the case of very young children, play routines can be among the best times to introduce communication devices and teach language and communication.

A substantial amount of preschool-level software has been developed to facilitate language and communication-skill development. Often this software can be used with very young children. *Choice Maker* by Microcomputers Systems for the Handicapped teaches making choices and scanning using a teaching hierarchy and environmental control. It pairs real objects, pictures, and computer graphics. Laureate's *First Words* builds vocabulary and labeling and also introduces and reinforces the concept of a scanning indicator. The *PEAL* (Programs for Early Acquisition of Language) software, developed by Laura Meyer and available through Don Johnston, uses the Muppet Learning Keys touchpad, real objects, and pictures to teach language and communication through play routines. Voice synthesizers are integral to all three programs.

Companies are beginning to develop communication and language-training programs for use with the TouchWindow, a device that mounts over the computer screen or on top of overlays and then allows the child to interact (using direct selection) with the computer by touching the window itself. *First Words* and *Talking Nouns I and II* and *Talking Verbs* by Laureate are available in TouchWindow versions. While they would be too advanced for most very young children, a creative practitioner could modify their overlays and thus make them usable by some children at the upper age range of this population. Project ACTT of the Macoomb Project has also developed programmable software called *Talking TouchWindow* that allows practitioners to develop their own courseware. Certainly this technology holds significant promise for very young children, and hopefully more programs will become available for it.

Software such as that described above is not intended to bear the sole responsibility for training young children to communicate. Communication is far too complex. What they are designed to do, however, is help practitioners structure good, creative, fun learning experiences for the children. To date, such support has not been available for use on the dedicated augmentative devices. Practitioners have developed all their own overlays and programs to meet their training needs. This situation may be changing, however.

Van Tatenhove[18] developed software for the Touch and Light Talkers that is appropriate for young children functioning cognitively and linguistically on a two- to three-year-old level. Currently being marketed by Prentke Romich Company, *Power in Play* focuses on the kinds of activities typically enjoyed by young children. The therapist can build communication interaction practice around these activities or themes as they are called. Picture-based overlays for each of the five themes accompany the software. In addition, each theme has three levels of difficulty. For example, the picture of the piano (piano icon) represents "Let's sing" at level 1, "Let's sing a song" at level 2, and "I like to make music—Let's sing a song" at level 3. One particularly needed overlay focuses on routine communication: Saying good morning and night to parents, telling them "I love you," and saying prayers. Other overlays include playing "Simon Says," having a treasure hunt, and playing rhyming games.

Today it is no longer argued whether using augmentative communication will prevent speech from developing. In fact, it can facilitate vocal communication.[9,19,20] Providing augmentative communication early provides a systematic means of shaping early communicative attempts into meaningful communication. Just as developing a language early has been shown to affect the subsequent communication abilities of deaf children,[21] offering very young nonverbal children with physical disabilities a way to communicate with their own "voices" may alter their subsequent abilities in reading and writing (B. Baker, personal communication, June 1988). Certainly it allows them to be heard.

Adapting microcomputers for very young handicapped children

Once children have the prerequisite skills necessary to operate toys, and particularly when they are using dedicated augmentative communication devices, they are better prepared to have more successful interactions with a microcomputer. Many of the augmentative communication devices noted above have some type of interface to commonly available microcomputers, enabling the child to use the communication device as an adapted keyboard. This has the advantage of not requiring the child to learn to use another adaptive device in order to use the computer.

If a child has not learned to use an augmentative communication device or is not able to use the device effectively with the computer, then it is important to use peripheral devices as alternatives to the keyboard. The keyboard is very busy, and young children are easily distracted or unable to focus on a limited selection of keys that activate the computer. Commonly available peripheral devices include touch monitors, adapted keyboards and touch pads, voice activation, and switch interfaces. The TouchWindow by Personal Touch is a touch-sensitive screen that is placed over the monitor. This screen allows the child to use direct selection, touching the monitor, to activate the software. Touch pads include the Muppet Learning Keys by Sunburst and the Power Pad by Dunamis. These pads can be modified into single or multiple switches and adapted keyboards. The Muppet Learning Keys, for example, have the alphabet in order as well as a ruler that illustrates numbers and a watercolor set for color selection. Switch interfaces vary from simple adapters for the computer game port to more sophisticated devices that act as keyboard emulators. Simple switch adapters require that the software be designed for single- or multiple-switch input. Keyboard emulators such as the PC Aid for the IBM and the Adaptive Firmware Card for the Apple II series do not require specialized software, since they emulate the keyboard input and put a scanning display at the bottom of the monitor. Thus a child can select the appropriate input (eg, A, B, or C) by pressing a switch when the indicator is on the letter.

Most of the software available for young children is for the Apple II series computers, although for children who need a portable computer, the IBM laptop or IBM-compatible computer with voice synthesis can provide a more appropriate technology. Software for microcomputers generally falls along traditional academic and readiness domains and uses color, graphics, animation, sound, and voice synthesis for this population. When introducing computers to very young handicapped children who have been exposed to the toys and switches noted previously, it is important to minimize the number of new concepts and skills. If switch-activated software is initially introduced, then the only new variables introduced will be screen graphics and in many cases sound or voice synthesis. For example, the Macoomb Project ACTT's *Master Blaster* and *Switch and See* use a switch activation to teach cause and effect. Laureate's *Creature Chorus* and *Creature Antics* also teach cause and effect with a single switch, but also introduce another variable, the touch screen, which allows a child to directly activate the computer graphic by touching the monitor screen. This assists a child who has difficulty understanding the relationship between pressing a switch and what happens on the computer monitor. As skill with the computer increases, there is also software that introduces scanning, such as *Rabbit Scanner* by Michael Rettig and Robert Greenlee (distributed by Don Johnston).

Development of language skills, discussed earlier, is one of the areas for which a substantial amount of preschool software is available. Other software is available for readiness activities such as matching, number recognition, letter recognition, and sound recognition but are at the high end of the continuum for the population discussed in this article. Examples of this type of software include *Stickybear ABCs* and *Stickybear Numbers* by Xerox. Software such as the *Motor Training Games* produced by the University of Washington is also available in the areas of perceptual-motor development. Finally, software is available for other learning and recreational activities. Even board game software such as *Rockets to the Moon* by the University of California at Los Angeles/Los Angeles Unified School District (UCLA/LAUSD) Microcomputer Software allows handicapped young children to participate in games appropriate for their age. Graphics software such as *Face Maker* by Spinnaker enables children to draw or to compose drawings from subcomponents. Musical software allows children to explore sounds and songs familiar to preschool curriculum, such as *Wheels on the Bus* and *This Is the Way We Wash Our Face* by UCLA/LAUSD. These programs use the Power Pad with special overlays to allow the child to make choices to sing different parts of these songs.

• • •

Introducing technology to very young children with disabilities is still quite early in its development. While there are many obvious potential benefits to early intervention using this technology, the state of the art is still not sufficiently advanced to enable professionals serving these children to meet the needs of this population easily or adequately. However, these children can be trained in many of the skills necessary for successful use of computer and augmentative communication technology without the use of expensive or complicated equipment. Thus, when they are physically and developmentally ready to use available technology, these children will be able to receive the maximum benefits that technology can make in quality of life and the ability to learn and become as independent as possible. The authors also expect that with the rapid advances in technology development, changes in state-of-the-art hardware and software will soon make appropriate technology available for younger children.

REFERENCES

1. Behrmann M: *Integrating Computers Into the Curriculum.* Boston, College-Hill Press, 1988.
2. Peterson N: *Early Intervention for Handicapped and At-Risk Children.* Denver, Love Publishing, 1987.
3. Brinker R, Lewis M: Making the world work with microcomputers: A learning prosthesis for handicapped infants. *Except Child* 1982;49(2):163–170.
4. Piaget J: *The Origins of Intelligence in Children.* London, International Universities Press, 1952.
5. Behrmann M, Lahm E: Babies and robots: Technology to assist learning. *Rehabil Lit* 1984;45(7–8):194–201.
6. Behrmann M, Lahm E: Critical learning: Multiply handicapped babies get on-line, in Behrmann M, Lahm E: *Proceedings of the National Conference on the Use of Microcomputers in Special Education.* Reston, Va, Council for Exceptional Children, 1984.
7. Marozas D, May D: Early intervention: How effective is it?, in Marozas D, May D (eds): *Issues and Practices in Special Education.* New York, Longman, 1988.
8. Porter L, Lahm E, Behrmann M, et al: Designing picture-based software for the cognitively young. *J Div Early Childhood* 1986;10(3):231–239.

9. Musselwhite C, St. Louis K: *Communication Programming for Persons with Severe Handicaps: Vocal and Augmentative Strategies,* ed 2. Boston, Little, Brown, 1988.
10. Mirenda P: Designing pictorial communication systems for physically able-bodied students with severe handicaps. *Augment Alternat Commun* 1985;1:58–64.
11. Lloyd J: Introduction to augmentative communication—Symbol systems. Seminar presentation, West Lafayette, Ind, Purdue University, Jul 31, 1987.
12. Hutinger P: *Activating Children Through Technology (ACTT) Curriculum.* Macoomb, Ill, Western Illinois University, 1986.
13. Wilds M: *The Future Role of Technology/Computers in the Pre-school Handicapped Classroom.* Read before the National Council for Exceptional Children Conference, Washington, DC, Mar 28, 1988.
14. Goosens' C, Crain S: *Augmentative Communication: Assessment Resource.* Wauconda, Ill, Don Johnston Developmental Equipment, 1986.
15. Goosens' C, Crain S: *Augmentative Communication: Intervention Resource.* Wauconda, Ill, Don Johnston Developmental Equipment, 1986.
16. Burkhardt L: *Homemade Battery Powered Toys and Educational Devices for Severely Handicapped Children.* College Park, Md, self-published, 1980.
17. Mittler J: Electronic toys and robots, in Behrmann M (ed): *Integrating Computers into the Curriculum.* Boston, College-Hill Press, 1988.
18. Van Tatenhove G: Teaching power through augmentative communication: Guidelines for early intervention. *J Childhood Commun Disord* 1987;10(2):185–199.
19. McCormick L, Shane H: Augmentative communication, in McCormick L, Schiefelbusch R (eds): *Early Language Intervention.* Columbus, Ohio, Charles E. Merrill, 1984.
20. McDonald E: Early identification and treatment of children at risk for speech development, in Schiefelbusch R (ed): *Nonspeech Language and Communication: Analysis and Intervention.* Austin, Tex, Pro-Ed, 1980.
21. Moores D: *Educating the Deaf: Psychology, Principles, and Practices.* Boston, Houghton Mifflin, 1978.

SUGGESTED READINGS

Burkhardt LJ: *Using Computers and Speech Synthesis to Facilitate Communicative Interaction with Young and/or Severely Handicapped Children.* College Park, Md, self-published, 1988.

Burkhardt LJ: *More Homemade Battery Devices for Severely Handicapped Children with Suggested Activities.* College Park, Md, self-published, 1988.

Charlebois-Marois C: *Everybody's Technology—A Sharing of Ideas in Augmentative Communication.* Montreal, Carlecoms, 1986.

Hutinger PL: *Activating Children Through Technology—Starter Kit.* Macoomb Ill, Project ACTT, Western Illinois University, 1986.

Wright C: *From Toys to Computers: Access for the Physically Disabled Child.* Wauconda, Ill, Don Johnston Developmental Equipment, 1987.

A comprehensive approach to using video for training infant and toddler caregivers

Peter L. Mangione, PhD
Senior Research Associate
Center for Child and Family Studies
Far West Laboratory for Educational Research and Development
San Francisco, California

IN 1986, approximately 50% of children under 3 years of age had mothers in the labor force.[1] The number of trained people available to provide high-quality child care pales in comparison to the number of infants and toddlers currently in care.[2] Moreover, training is not easy for many of the existing providers to obtain. Most of them are family day care providers who work long hours and have little time and limited resources to seek training. Yet adequate training of staff in early development and care has been consistently found to be a critical ingredient in the quality of child care programs.[3,4]

Concerned about the quality of available infant care, the California State Department of Education's Child Development Division (CDD) initiated the development of a comprehensive training system for both center-based and home-based providers of group care to infants and toddlers. It selected Far West Laboratory for Educational Research and Development (FWL) to develop this system.

The purpose of this development work was twofold: first, to create a training system that could be used by California's Child Development Division in its efforts to facilitate the training of infant and toddler caregivers who work in its subsidized programs; and second, to produce comprehensive video and written training materials that could be integrated into caregiver training activities throughout the United States. Since many caregivers are not college educated, the materials had to be geared to a secondary level of education. And in light of increasing numbers of infant and toddler caregivers in the United States who are non-English speaking, CDD decided that the materials should be created in Chinese and Spanish in addition to English. Work on the Program for Infant/Toddler Caregivers began at FWL in 1986 under the direction of Dr J. Ronald Lally. Development work has proceeded as a close collaboration between FWL and CDD.

This article provides an overview of California's effort to promote large-scale training of infant and toddler caregivers. It documents preliminary steps that have led to the articulation of a set of guidelines for creating a series of training videos. An effort to disseminate video training materials on a pilot basis is summarized as

The author acknowledges the contributions of Dr J. Ronald Lally to this article and his leadership in the development of the project described herein. Other key contributors to the project are Sheila Signer, Program Associate, Far West Laboratory for Educational Research and Development, Dr Robert Servantes, Assistant Superintendent, Janet Poole, Assistant Director, and Mary Smithberger, Consultant, Child Development Division, California State Department of Education.
Support for the project has come from the California State Department of Education, Child Development Division, the Carnegie Corporation and the Harris Foundation.

Inf Young Children 1990; 3(1): 61–68

well. Lastly, plans to develop both training workshops and guides for trainers are briefly described.

PRELIMINARY STEPS

Rationale for using video

The centerpiece of the Program for Infant/Toddler Caregivers is a series of training videos that is supplemented by various written materials, most notably a series of guides on infant toddler caregiving. Several considerations influenced the decision by the program's developers to make videotaped material central in the training system. Above all, becoming a sensitive observer of young children is an essential part of learning about how to care for them appropriately and effectively. Without guidance, an untrained observer can miss many subtle aspects of an infant's behavior. Videotaped material can be highlighted with both visual effects and narration to draw the attention of viewers to subtleties of infant behavior and help them become more sensitive observers.

Another consideration underlying the choice of video is that high-quality training materials can be made available to large numbers of child care providers. Videotaped programs are becoming increasingly transportable and can be broadcast over public and private networks. Finally, if made well, videos can both inform and inspire the viewer. A video that shows quality care being provided to young children can both engage the interest of caregivers and present positive role models to them.

Review of materials

Finding out precisely what kind of media training materials, including video, were currently available for infant and toddler caregivers was considered necessary before moving ahead with production of an entire series of videos. Honig and Wittmer[5] compiled information from a review of 91 media training materials for infant and toddler caregivers in an annotated guide. This guide provides information on the format of each program (eg, video or film), the topics it covers, the language in which it is presented, and its cost. In addition, Honig and Wittmer[5] rated the audiovisual quality, accuracy, and usefulness of each program and judged its appropriateness for various audiences (eg, caregivers, parents, advanced college students).

Although most of the materials identified by Honig and Wittmer in their search are either for parents or for college-level students of human development, much of the information in them is useful to caregivers. But these materials rarely address questions related to caring for infants in groups. Thus, such topics as designing environments for groups of infants, group size, age mixture of infants in groups, individual variation within a group, and dealing with parental concerns and needs receive little treatment in currently available media training materials.

The review by Honig and Wittmer[5] also revealed that training videos that are available come from various sources, their costs vary greatly, their content tends to be general, the topics they cover often overlap, and few are in languages other than English. These factors contribute to the piecemeal use of videos in the training of infant and toddler caregivers. Against this background, the number of training videos being made on topics related to group care has recently increased. The video project described herein is part of the growing recognition of the need to support the training of center-based and family child care providers. It represents an attempt to provide a comprehensive series of training videos in English, Spanish, and Chinese, with each covering a specific topic and all of them grounded in a common approach to caring for young children.

Needs assessment

Survey data were gathered from 405 child care providers in the State of California (278 center-based, 127 family child care providers) to document their perceived needs for training.[6] The questionnaire focused on three issues: content needs, approaches to learning, and the context for viewing training videos. Caregivers were first asked to rank video topics according to their need for information. Over 50% of the questionnaire respondents ranked the topic "Setting Up a Safe and Interesting Environment" among their top five choices of videos they would find useful to view. Other topics that frequently received high rankings were in the domain of social-emotional growth and socialization. These findings were used to establish priorities in the development of the videos and related written guides.

Caregivers were also asked to rank the effectiveness of different means of learning about early development and care. The respondents ranked options including "Talking with a Colleague," "Attending a Lecture," "Participating in a Group Discussion," "Reading," "Observing a Master Caregiver in Action," and "Experimenting and Seeing What Works." The option that was most often ranked among the top five ranks was "Observing a Master Caregiver in Action." This result strengthened the view that observation is an important mode of learning for students of early development and care.

Finally, respondents ranked the desirability of various contexts or settings for viewing a training video on infant care. They were found to favor settings in which a trainer and peers are present. Opportunities to ask questions of a specialist as well as to discuss the content of a video in a group were identified as vital to their learning. This result held true for both center-based and family child care providers. In addition, the subsample of family child care providers, who conceivably would have a more difficult time finding substitutes and arranging for transportation to training sessions, gave high rankings to the option of viewing a video alone at home. Nevertheless, the general interest of caregivers in opportunities for discussion with a trainer or specialist indicated that presenting information via video should be integrated into a comprehensive training system.

Guidelines for quality care

The Program for Infant/Toddler Caregivers represents an intensive effort to develop high-quality training materials whose focus is the care of young children in group settings. The philosophical core guiding the creation of the program's video and written materials centers around infants' need for warm, supportive relationships with their caregivers. Both a close relationship between caregiver and child and conditions that foster the development of a sense of security, confidence, and identity in the child are essential to quality care. Moreover, quality care springs from a compassionate understanding of development and respect for each child as an individual with personal needs and inclinations. The formative role of family history and culture in the lives of infants and toddlers and their parents is also considered important. Establishing a partnership with parents based on sensitivity and respect is a vital part of caring for young children.

The program addresses every aspect of group care (eg, environment, caregiving routines) within the above philosophical approach. (The full range of content covered in its first four training modules is shown in the box.) In order for the program to evolve coherently, a foundation was laid in the form of a statement of guidelines for quality care. National and state experts, both researchers and practitioners, contributed directly to the creation of the document "Visions for Infant/Toddler Care: Guidelines for Professional Caregiving."[7] CDD participated extensively in the creation of this document. The guidelines defined in the "Visions" document have become the guidelines for the State's infant and toddler programs and the basis of its infant and toddler program quality review instrument. This instrument, which is used in agency evaluations of state-subsidized infant and toddler group care programs, is designed for use by any infant and toddler program interested in assessing the quality of care it provides.

ATTRIBUTES OF THE VIDEOS

Information derived from the review of media materials, the needs assessment, and the articulation of guidelines for quality infant care provided a framework for the development of the training videos. Advice and recommendations to the project team from the program's national and state advisors, video production ex-

The First Four Training Modules of the Program for Infant/Toddler Caregivers

Module I: Social Emotional Growth and Socialization
Infant/Toddler Caregiving: A Guide to Social-Emotional Growth & Socialization
Videos and video magazines:
First Moves: Welcoming a Child to a New Caregiving Setting
Getting in Tune: Establishing Relationships with Infants and Toddlers
Flexible, Fearful or Feisty: The Temperaments of Infants and Toddlers

Module II: Group Care
Infant/Toddler Caregiving: A Guide to Routines
Infant/Toddler Caregiving: A Guide to Setting up the Environment
Videos and video magazines:
It's Not Just Routine: Feeding, Diapering and Napping Infants and Toddlers
Respectfully Yours: Magda Gerber's Approach to Professional Infant/Toddler Care
Caring for Infants in Groups (working title)
Space to Grow: Creating a Child Care Environment for Infants and Toddlers

Module III: Learning and Development
Infant/Toddler Caregiving: A Guide to Intellectual Development and Creativity
Infant/Toddler Caregiving: A Guide to Language Development and Communication
Videos and video magazines:
Discoveries in Infancy: Cognitive Development and Creativity (working title)
Early Messages: Communicating With Infants (working title)
The Ages of Infancy: Caring for Young, Mobile and Older Infants

Module IV: Culture, Family, and Providers
Infant/Toddler Caregiving: A Guide to Culturally Sensitive Care
Infant/Toddler Caregiving: A Guide to Creating Partnerships with Parents
Videos and video magazines:
A World of Difference: Culturally Sensitive Care for Infants and Toddlers (working title)
Sharing the Care: Parent–Provider Relationships in Infant–Toddler Care (working title)

perts, caregiver trainers, and practitioners helped shape the content and style of the videos. This input influenced such characteristics as the length of the videos, the extent to which theory is covered *v* practical suggestions, the breadth of material presented, and the type of effects used in the videos.

For several reasons, a length of 25 to 30 minutes was considered to be optimal for the videos. Advisors representing public television systems recommended this length because it would make the videos suitable for programming in one-half hour time slots. Keeping the attention of the viewers was an additional concern. The longer a video, the more likely it is to lose the audience's attention. Nevertheless, a video has to be long enough so that learning can be reinforced through repeated exposure to the concepts being covered. In other words, time is needed to introduce a video's major concepts, treat them in detail, and then review them. A video of no more than 30 minutes in length also gives a trainer flexibility in integrating it into a larger workshop.

Experts in video production advised that each video should be narrow in scope, covering only a limited number of concepts. Since as a series the videos were intended to constitute a comprehensive package, each could focus on a specific topic. However, to be handled adequately, a narrowly defined video topic must be treated in considerable detail.

In light of these competing concerns, the approach adopted was to give ample coverage to a small number of concepts, while trying not to overdo the presentation of any given concept. In effect, the concepts themselves organized the information presented in a video. This type of structure facilitates trainers' using part of a video to concentrate on a specific concept without having to show trainees the entire video. For example, one of the concepts dealt with in the video "Space to Grow: Creating a Child Care Environment for Infants and Toddlers" is flexibility. If a trainer wanted to focus solely on flexibility during a training session, the section of the video that addresses this aspect of environmental design could be preselected for viewing and discussion.

Another consideration in making the videos was striking a balance between developmental theory and research and practical guidelines and suggestions. The advisory groups strongly recommended creating videos that are practical in nature. Following this advice, the videos introduce background material on early development and then spell out practical tips and recommendations based on theory and practice. Much of the theory and research on the development of young children and related practical advice refers to caregiving by parents in the child's home. This material has been adapted to the context of group care and supplemented by knowledge derived from group care practice.

The Program's video "Flexible, Fearful or Feisty: The Temperaments of Infants and Toddlers" exemplifies how information from theory and research can be applied to the group care context. The video begins by briefly identifying Thomas and Chess' nine indicators of temperament as described by Chess.[8] These indicators are then used to define three major temperament types and illustrate the effect of group care on each of these types. Ideas and suggestions are then offered on how to deal with the sometimes competing demands of children of different temperament types in a group.

One of the challenges in making videos on infant care is finding ways to convey the subtle aspects of quality caregiving. Critically analyzing each scene before deciding what to communicate about it has become an essential part of the process of creating each video. The analysis stage often consists of repeated viewing of a sequence and discussion among the project team on how to interpret both the caregiver's and the children's behavior. A thorough analysis results in the development of simple, direct language to draw attention to the key aspects of the scene and gives insight into the kinds of editing techniques and visual effects that would effectively highlight the points made in the narration. One of the scenes in the video "Getting in Tune: Creating Nurturing Relationships with Infants and Toddlers" illustrates how the combination of video editing and simple, direct narration can communicate the subtlety of interaction between caregivers and infants. The scene of a caregiver and two young children is first shown completely through while the narration highlights the generally respectful manner of the caregiver. The viewer is then invited to take a second look at the scene. This time the sequence is stopped at key points, and the narration describes how the caregiver subtly redirects the behavior of one child whose play is starting to upset the other child. Other techniques that have been useful in illumination content have included showing sequences in slow motion and highlighting certain parts of the screen.

In order to engage the interest of caregivers, the videos emphasize the rewarding aspects of infant caregiving as well as acknowledge its challenges and difficulties. The videos visually and verbally communicate young children's need for warm and trusting relationships with their caregivers. Examples of the natural enjoyment of the relationship shared by caregiver and child are shown throughout the series of videos. Infants and toddlers make new discoveries about themselves and their world on a daily basis, and this process can be fascinating to adults. The videos present sequences that strengthen this fascination in caregivers. Humor is used in the videos to convey the light and playful side of infant caregiving. A respectful tone is conveyed in the videos, and the importance of responsive caregiving to young children is underscored. In other words, the style of presentation in the videos is intended to recognize and honor the profession of infant and toddler caregiving.

While placing emphasis on the rewarding side of caregiving, the videos also address its challenges and difficulties. Caring for young children is demanding work and can often be stressful. Child care providers have to deal with, among other things, parents' concerns and needs, scheduling issues, various regulations, special contingencies like sick or injured children, running a business, and children who exhibit difficult behavior. When addressing sources of stress for caregivers in the videos and other training materials, the problems are recognized and suggestions are offered that, if put into practice, may help moderate the stressfulness of a situation. This approach reflects the primary purpose of the videos, that is, to give caregivers the tools they need to nurture and support the development of children in their care.

DISSEMINATION OF THE VIDEOS

As the first videos of the Program for Infant/Toddler Caregivers have become available, several dissemination activities are occurring simultaneously. These activities include the study of three pilot video resource centers, the development of training institutes for trainers, and the creation of guide materials for trainers. In effect, the primary dissemination strategy underlying these activities is to build on established training efforts. Trainers who become adept at using the program's materials will be able to communicate effectively about the program with colleagues and organizations interested in promoting caregiver training and present the materials to increasing numbers of caregivers in need of training. In addition, the videos thus far completed are being distributed by the California State Department of Education and being shown as a series on public television in parts of California.

Video resource centers

CDD has established three caregiver training resource centers in different regions on a pilot basis. The local child care resource and referral agencies in each of the areas house the training video resources. The resource centers' inventories include copies of the first four program videos, the annotated guide to media training materials, the visions of infant and toddler caregiving document, and a draft copy of "Infant/Toddler Caregiving: A Guide to Social-Emotional Growth and Socialization." In addition, numerous other videos and books round out the collection of training materials.

The purpose in setting up the training resource centers was twofold: first, to document how video and written training materials are used at the local level, and second, to discover ways to facilitate the use of video materials by trainers in their training activities. Data are being gathered on, among other things, who checks out the videos (eg, trainers, program directors, individual caregivers) and where the videos are being viewed (eg, in training workshops, at centers, in homes). In addition, trainers and community college instructors who use the materials in their work are being interviewed about the usefulness of the materials and strategies for supporting training activities for infant and toddler caregivers.

The evaluation of pilot dissemination through local training resource centers is currently in progress. Anecdotal information gathered during systematic data collection is pointing to two major factors in the use of video materials in training. First, the more accessible materials are, the more likely trainers and caregivers are to use them. One of the most successful attempts to make the videos more available has been the implementation of a delivery service. In response to numerous complaints about the limited hours of operation of one of the video resource centers, the sponsoring agency hired a high school student whose job it is to deliver videos to people interested in using them. Second, trainers are reporting a need for guidance and support materials to facilitate their using video materials in caregiver training activities. Both of these factors correspond to findings reported in the literature on the distribution and use of instructional media materials.[9]

Training institutes for trainers

One of the strategies for supporting caregiver training efforts is the development of institutes for trainers. The purpose of the institutes is both to give trainers the opportunity to explore in depth the content of the program's video and written materials and to help them integrate the videos with the instructional techniques they use in training (eg, lectures, small group activities). Institute participants are provided an overview of major content areas of infant and toddler caregiving; information drawn from current theory, research, and practice forms the backbone of this overview.

Detailed study of a set of videos complements the survey of content areas. As stated above, the videos are also considered with respect to the instructional context in which they are presented. Such issues as whether to show only parts of a particular video, how to treat a topic in greater depth than a video does, or how to address controversies stirred up by a video receive attention. This kind of intensive study of the program's materials promotes their use as a comprehensive series of videos and written documents as an alternative to using each of the materials in a piecemeal fashion.

Support materials for trainers

Another strategy for supporting trainers is the development of video and written materials that provide ideas and suggestions related to using the program's videos. Two videos will be created. One of them will show a sampling of scenes from the program's videos; trainers will be able to gain a sense of both the video series as a whole and the content and style of each particular video. This information is intended to help trainers plan how they will use the series. A second video will focus on how to use the program's videos to train infant and toddler caregivers. It will, among other things, demonstrate a training session that is organized around showing a video. An underlying theme will be using video material to foster the development of the observational skills of training participants.

The written guide for trainers will treat each of the program's videos in a separate section. Each of these sections will offer ideas and suggestions for using the video in training. Content issues raised by a video and points for discussion will be covered in each section as well. Different approaches to presenting particular video material will be highlighted in the guide. For example, certain sequences in a video may be especially interesting to view a second time after discussion. The guide will also address how to adapt each video to the training needs of different groups (eg, caregivers of children with special needs). Finally, the guide will present the complete training system, specifying how videos and written materials fit into training modules and can be used in combination with each other.

In sum, the development of a comprehensive approach to large-scale training of infant and toddler caregivers is a complex task. Attention must be given to such issues as training needs, the selection of content, the style and technical quality of training materials, and dissemination strategies. As the program has evolved, dissemination has become as important as product development. Now that a good portion of the program's videos are available, the greatest challenge is to continue to find ways to integrate them into efforts around the country to promote the training of infant and toddler caregivers.

As the Program for Infant/Toddler Caregiver's videos and written training have been completed, they are being published and distributed by the California State Department of Education. These materials are available for purchase from: California State Department of Education, Bureau of Publications, Sales Unit, P.O. Box 271, Sacramento, CA 95802-0271.

REFERENCES

1. *Infants can't wait: The numbers.* Washington, DC: National Center for Clinical Infant Programs; 1986.
2. Hofferth SL. What is the demand and supply of child care in the United States? *Young Child.* 1989;44:28–33.
3. Howes C. Relations between child care and schooling. *Dev Psychol.* 1988;24:53–57.
4. Whitebook M, Howes C, Phillips D. *Who cares? Child care teachers and the quality of care in America.* Oakland, Calif: Child Care Employee Project; 1989.
5. Honig AS, Wittmer DS. *Infant/toddler caregiving: An annotated guide to media training materials.* Sacramento, Calif: California State Department of Education; 1988.
6. Mangione PL. An assessment of training needs of infant and toddler caregivers in California (technical report). San Francisco, Calif: Far West Laboratory; 1986.
7. *Visions for Infant/Toddler Care: Guidelines for Professional Caregiving.* Sacramento, Calif: California State Department of Education; 1988.
8. Chess S. Temperaments of infants and toddlers. In: Lally JR, ed. *Infant/Toddler Caregiving: A Guide to Social Emotional Growth and Socialization.* Sacramento, Calif: California State Department of Education. In press.
9. Cambre MA. A reappraisal of instructional television. Syracuse, NY: Educational Resources Information Center, 1987.

Early intervention for technology-dependent infants and young children

Elizabeth Ahmann, RN, ScD
Consultant
Washington, DC

Kathleen A. Lipsi, MA, EdS
Developmental Specialist
Department of Neonatology
Children's National Medical Center
Washington, DC

ESTIMATES OF the number of technology-dependent children currently cared for at home are difficult to arrive at and uncertain at best. In 1987, the Office of Technology Assessment published the prevalence estimates indicated in Table 1. Although not all technology-dependent children are in the 0 to 3-year age range, increased survival of very low birth weight infants seems to be the greatest contributor to increases in the technology-dependent population.[1]

Public Law 99-457 emphasizes the importance of early intervention services for infants and young children who have developmental delays. This law also encourages states to extend early intervention services to infants and young children at risk for delays, to those who are chronically ill, and to those who require frequent or lengthy hospital stays.[2,3] As states extend their services, early intervention programs will face the challenge of providing appropriate treatment to the growing population of technology-dependent children.

For the most part, general principles regarding the planning, implementation, and evaluation of early intervention treatment programs can be applied to the population of technology-dependent infants and young children with certain modifications. This article highlights these modifications and addresses key issues and specific skills relevant to intervention with this population.

A discussion of the factors influencing the choice of the most appropriate setting for early intervention services for technology-dependent children is beyond the scope of this article. Nonetheless, many of the issues and strategies addressed in this article may be applied in a variety of intervention programs and settings. The planning, intervention, and evaluation of early intervention services for technology-dependent infants and young children is illustrated here using the example of technology-dependent infants with bronchopulmonary dysplasia (BPD). Considerations will be similar for children with other diagnoses, and many of the treatment considerations are also applicable to the medically fragile child who is not technology dependent.

The authors thank Anne B. Jeschke, RPT, and Connie Lierman, RN, MSN, of Children's National Medical Center for their thoughtful reviews of the draft manuscript.

Inf Young Children 1991; 3(4): 67–77

Table 1. Summary of OTA estimates of the size of the technology-dependent child population, 1987

Defined population	*Estimated number of children*
Group 1	
Requires ventilator assistance	680–2,000
Group 2	
Requires parenteral nutrition	350–700
Requires prolonged intravenous drugs	270–8,275
Group 3	
Requires other device-based respiratory or nutrition support	1,000–6,000
Rounded subtotal (1 + 2 + 3)	2,300–17,000
Group 4	
Requires apnea monitoring	6,800–45,000
Requires renal dialysis	1,000–6,000
Requires other device-associated nursing	Unknown, perhaps 30,000 or more

Source: U.S. Office of Technology Assessment. *Technology Dependent Children: Hospital v. Home Care—A Technical Memorandum.* Washington, DC: Government Printing Office; 1987:4. Publication no. OTA-TM-H-38.

PLANNING A TREATMENT PROGRAM

Planning an early intervention program for technology-dependent children involves setting both short- and long-term goals and objectives based on a thorough assessment of the needs of the child and family. It requires close coordination among multiple care providers.

Child needs

The child's medical needs are a primary consideration in planning a developmental treatment program. As a first step, the early interventionist must obtain documentation of the child's medical status and the limitations it may place on therapeutic interventions. (It is recognized that early intervention services are provided by various disciplines. For that reason, the generic term "interventionist" will be used here.) Factors to consider include the child's respiratory condition, neurologic status, and tolerance for positioning and activity. Medications or other treatments, the schedule of administration, and their effect on the child's state and endurance should be noted. The interventionist also needs an orientation to normal physiologic and autonomic responses for the individual child. Finally, the establishment of realistic goals and objectives for development must be based on a consideration of both the child's functional level and the adjusted age level for the premature infant.[4,5]

Early interventionists must be familiar with the constraints associated with technology dependence and ways the therapy plan can be adapted to accommodate the need for medical equipment. Table 2 lists issues to consider. Technology dependence coupled with long hospital stays often limits the child's sensory-motor experience and thereby interferes with the normal process of development.[6]

Table 2. An overview of developmental issues in high-technology home care: Age 0–3 years

Developmental stage	*Developmental issues*	*Interventions*
Infant (0–1 year)	Sensory experience	Encourage tactile and verbal instructions
		Provide visual and auditory stimulation as tolerated
	Motor experience	Vary positioning to encourage freedom of movement
	Development of trust	Support parents in efforts to consistently meet infant's needs
		Encourage close relationship with one caregiver
	Oral–motor experience	Encourage nonnutritive sucking if necessary and tolerated
Toddler (1–3 years)	Development of autonomy	
	Freedom of mobility	Arrange equipment to facilitate mobility (eg, long oxygen tubing)
		When mobility must be restricted, provide suitable alternate activities (eg, reading a story, playing with blocks)
	Opportunity to explore	Provide safe environment (eg, cover electric outlets, secure knobs and dials on equipment)
	Oppositional behavior	Allow as much control as possible (eg, child can hold saline during suctioning)
		Do not offer choice when there is none
	Development of language	Provide simple explanation
		Repetition is necessary
		Assist tracheotomized ventilator-dependent child with alternate expressive modality

Adapted with permission from An Overview of Developmental Issues in Pediatric High-Tech Home Care © 1990, Elizabeth Ahmann, ScD.

The treatment program should be designed to address these deficits and avoid further detrimental effects. Additionally, because technology-dependent children lie still and can get very stiff, apparent limitations in active movement are often limitations in passive movement (Jeschke AB. June 1990. Personal communication). In planning care, the interdisciplinary team should consider the need for basic physical therapy positions and activities appropriate to the child's needs.

Family needs

Family needs and concerns strongly influence the development of treatment programs for technology-dependent infants or young children. Family assessment is a complex issue, and careful consideration regarding both purpose and methods is required to obtain accurate and useful data.[7] Stages of adaptation, individual family coping mechanisms, and common themes for families with chronically ill and technology-dependent children should inform the assessment process.[8–11]

Parents should be considered an integral part of the assessment, planning, and evaluation team as detailed in the box, "Guidelines for Inclusion of Families." Because parents generally know their child best, they are an important source of knowledge for the interventionist regarding the child's abilities, limits, and signs of stress.[12] As the child's primary caretakers, parents also should be trained to follow through with aspects of the child's therapy on a regular basis. To minimize parental burden of care, recommendations should emphasize activities that can be incorporated into existing child and family routines.[3] The use of photographs or even videos can be helpful in reinforcing home programming suggestions,[13] and ongoing communication with family members can be encouraged through the use of a notebook or logbook updated regularly by all parties. Finally, in consideration of the many demands on the time of families of technology-dependent children, the interventionist should schedule home visits at the family's convenience, coordinate services with other care providers, and respect the family's need for privacy.[12,14–16] Additional guidelines for family-centered care are available from several sources.[14,17]

Service coordination

Coordination among service providers ensures that the child receives the most appropriate services and that duplication of services, conflicting treatment goals and recommendations, and excess family burden are avoided.[18]

Coordination of the multiple agencies and disciplines that may be involved in the care of a technology-dependent child requires a flexible team design. Initially, many technology-dependent children benefit most from a transdisciplinary approach that uses one or two key disciplines to address the child's primary

Guidelines for Inclusion of Families in the Planning and Delivery of Early Intervention Services

Concentrate on family priorities as perceived by families.
Respect parents' goals for the infant.
Include parents as primary members of the infant's assessment team.
Include parents in the planning of specific objectives and activities.
Develop activities to share knowledge about normal and delayed child development when appropriate.
Reinforce the observational skills of family members.
Explain all suggested activities and procedures so that families can generalize from specific knowledge.
Deal positively, not judgmentally, with all family members and encourage them to deal positively with the child.
Give positive feedback to families about specific achievements and encourage family members to recognize small increments of child's success.
Recognize and respect the diversity of cultural values.

Reprinted with permission from Kelly JF, Barnard KE. Early intervention. In: Wallace HM, Ryan G, Oglesby AC, eds. *Maternal and Child Health Practices,* 3rd ed. Oakland, Calif: Third Party Publishing; 1988, p. 653.

needs.[19,20] For example, the interventionist might train the nurse in essential aspects of therapy for a particular child. In a home-based program, the interventionist could then make fewer home visits while the nurse implements the therapy objectives and programming with the family. The interventionist is kept informed of the child's progress and remains available for consultation until the child can tolerate an increase in both service providers and frequency of treatment.

Regardless of team design, time and resources are best invested when the interventionist works closely with a nurse, particularly in the early stages of intervention. The nurse assists parents in orienting the interventionist to the child's condition, needs, and abilities; in developing an awareness of the child's limits and signs of stress; and in understanding the purpose of and safety precautions related to the child's medical equipment.

The interventionist who has no experience working with technology-dependent children should set up an informal mentoring or training program with an interventionist or therapist who has experience in treating and monitoring the care of this population.

IMPLEMENTING A TREATMENT PROGRAM

To implement a treatment program, the interventionist must be knowledgeable about the child's medical diagnosis and its implications for treatment. The interventionist also must be familiar with the child's medical equipment and strategies for working within the constraints posed by the equipment.

Diagnostic considerations

Bronchopulmonary dysplasia, the example used here, causes complex changes in the lungs of newborn infants after prolonged mechanical ventilation. Contributing factors appear to include prematurity, positive pressure ventilation, oxygen toxicity, pulmonary edema, increased airway resistance, and lung damage resulting from respiratory distress syndrome.[21-23] BPD has widely varied courses and a wide range of severity depending on the infant. Only a relatively small population of infants with BPD remain technology dependent beyond the period of their initial hospitalization.[1] Those who remain technology dependent generally have several components to their pulmonary disease, remain highly susceptible to infection, tire easily, and grow poorly.[21-25] Development in the infant with BPD may be delayed for any of several reasons: poor nutritional status; inadequate sensory stimulation resulting from extended hospital stays, mechanical ventilation, and isolation in oxygen tents; and other perinatal and neonatal events.[23,26,27]

Before the interventionist treats an infant or young child with BPD, observing the child's physiologic and developmental status at rest is essential.[28,29] The interventionist should carefully observe the child's respiratory rate and pattern, look for nasal flaring and retractions, examine the child's skin color, and observe both resting muscle tone and state. Asking a parent to hold and play with the child gives the interventionist an opportunity for further observation (Jeschke AB. April 1990. Personal communication). Parents can then be asked to take the child through a specific series of positions and activities to give the interventionist a more comprehensive assessment of the child's tolerance for type and degree of stimulation and for positioning, endurance, and recovery period after activity.

The infant or young child with BPD may be easily overtaxed and the interventionist should become familiar with the child's individual stress signals, which can include the following:

- chest retractions (intercostal and suprasternal),
- nasal flaring,
- marked increase in respiratory rate,
- difficulty returning to resting respiratory rate,
- increased heart rate,
- increased duskiness or mottling of skin color,
- clammy appearance,
- flailing of limbs,
- change in muscle tone,
- tremors,

- hiccoughs,
- defecation,
- excessive crying, and
- persistent gaze aversion.[28,30]

Als's[31] theory of synactive organizational behavior development emphasizes the importance of assessing and interpreting autonomic, motoric, state, and attention-interaction responses as an infant's means of communicating distress. Some stress may be tolerable if recovery to the normal baseline is rapid, but the interventionist should avoid overtaxing the child. Treatment sessions should be planned at the time of day the child is most rested, has not just eaten, and is not otherwise stressed. The interventionist should adjust the length of treatment sessions as appropriate and allow rest periods during the sessions. Feedback from parents about the child's recovery period after each treatment session will assist the interventionist in gauging the effects of the interventions.

Technology considerations

Infants or young children with BPD may be dependent on or assisted by one or more types of medical equipment. The interventionist should be familiar with the following types of equipment: suction machine, apnea monitor, oxygen delivery system, and mechanical ventilation system. A tracheostomy may be present. Personnel in the early intervention program should be trained in both routine and emergency care procedures relevant to the individual child's needs and equipment, particularly if other trained caregivers will not be present.[32,33]

A suction machine assists the child in clearing secretions. A suction machine or portable suction trap should always be available for children with a tracheostomy. Some children may also require oral and nasal suctioning. The need for suctioning may increase during activity, and the interventionist should be aware of the following indications for suctioning:

- secretions fill the oropharynx, nasopharynx, or tracheostomy tube;
- secretions increase in amount of thickness;
- fluids are audible as the infant breathes;
- the infant exhibits signs of respiratory distress such as retractions, flaring, grunting, or increased respiratory rate;
- the infant becomes pale or grey around the mouth or nose; and
- in an infant with a tracheostomy tube, breath sounds are dry and wheezy or are bubbly.[23,34]

The parent, nurse, or other trained individual should be summoned to suction the child as needed.

An apnea monitor, or cardiorespiratory monitor, may be used when there is a family history of sudden infant death syndrome, documented apnea, respiratory compromise of other causes, or tracheostomy and when a back-up alarm is needed during mechanical ventilation.[23,35] The monitor is attached to the infant via an electrode belt or patches, and an alarm sounds when breathing ceases for longer than a preset interval. Most monitors also have an alarm for low and high heart rates.

Many infants do not need to be attached to the monitor during therapy sessions. Since detachment allows for greater freedom during therapy treatment sessions, the interventionist should raise this question with the infant's parents and the managing physician.

Documented cases of electrical injury, including electrocution, have occurred because of misuse of apnea monitor components.[36] For this reason, interventionists not thoroughly familiar with the proper use of monitors should not connect or disconnect monitor components from each other or from the child without assistance. For the same reason, bathing and water play should be avoided when the child is attached to the monitor. When used properly, however, the monitor does not present any risk to the child or the interventionist.

Oxygen may be required for children with BPD. Children who require oxygen therapy need it during treatment sessions, and some children may require an increased flow rate before and during activity. If the child becomes pale or grey or exhibits signs of respiratory distress during or after services, the possibility of increased oxygen flow during the intervention sessions should be discussed with the physician.

A child with a tracheostomy generally uses a tracheostomy mask because it provides a directed flow of oxygen into the airway. Treatment sessions for a child without a tracheostomy can best be conducted if a nasal catheter or nasal cannula rather than a hood or tent is used. The catheter stays in place fairly well and delivers oxygen directly into the nares. A nasal cannula may roll during activity but can be held in place by a headband, Velcro straps, tape, or a clear surgical adhesive dressing (eg, Opsite or Tegaderm).[23] The prongs of most cannulas do not fit the nares of a small infant and can be clipped off.[37] Additionally, small holes cut around the cannula will make oxygen available even if the cannula slips or rolls (Fig 1).[23] "Blow-by" oxygen, where wide tubing is hand-held near the infant, is an alternative for infants requiring low concentrations during feeding or other activities. If the infant's current method of oxygen delivery unduly restricts treatment options, alternatives can be discussed with the family, physician, and respiratory therapist.

The length of tubing attached to the oxygen mask, catheter, or cannula is another factor to consider. Voyles[38] reported successfully using tubing of 6 to 30 feet to allow the oxygen-dependent child greater mobility. Because the length of tubing can affect the amount of oxygen the child receives, the physician and respiratory therapist should be consulted before changes are made.

The interventionist also should note that although oxygen itself is not combustible, it does cause sparks or flames to burn hotter and more rapidly. Because of

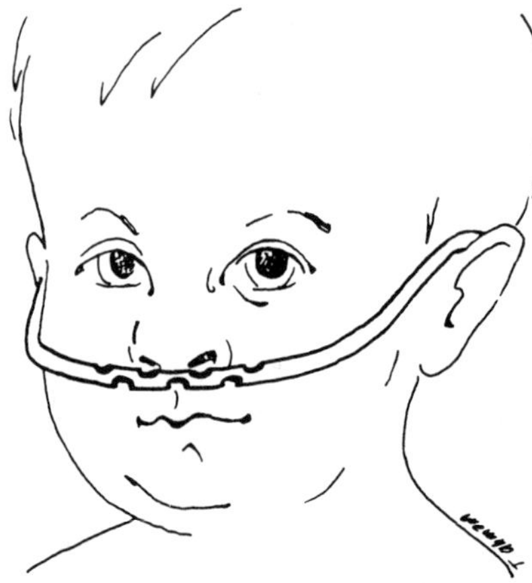

Fig 1. Perforated nasal cannula for oxygen delivery. Artwork courtesy of Teresa Ahmann. © 1985.

this, the following should be kept away from the oxygen source: electrical appliances and devices; cigarettes, sparks, and fire; alcohol-containing products; petroleum jelly or other petroleum-based products; and aerosols.[39] Nurses, respiratory therapists, and parents should be aware of additional safety precautions, which are reviewed in other sources.

Mechanical ventilation improves gas exchange in the lungs of infants and young children with severe BPD. Children may also require mechanical ventilation for a range of other respiratory and neuromuscular conditions.

Most children requiring mechanical ventilation for BPD have a positive pressure ventilator, which requires an endotracheal tube or, at home, a tracheostomy tube. The ventilator tube is attached to this artificial airway, and the lungs are inflated by increasing the pressure above the airway atmospheric pressure. Frates et al[35] and Dougherty[40] provide valuable information about negative pressure ventilation.

Children with BPD vary in their requirements for mechanical ventilation. Some require no ventilatory assistance, others require assistance for some part of the day or at night, and still others require assistance 24 hours a day. Before initiating a developmental program, the interventionist should discuss with the family and physician whether the child will require mechanical ventilation during treatment sessions.

Infants on mechanical ventilation spend a great deal of time in supine and side-lying positions. There is generally no contraindication to repositioning in semiupright or prone positions, however, and repositioning can be beneficial. An infant seat may be useful for semiupright positioning[6] and a blanket or sheet on the floor can be used to work in prone positions.

When the treatment area is laid out appropriately so that the ventilator tubing has adequate slack, there is generally no contraindication to moving the infant around during the treatment session. If the length of the tubing or the location of the ventilator in relation to the treatment area inhibits appropriate treatment, changes in these factors should be discussed with the parent and respiratory therapist. When moving and repositioning the ventilator-dependent child, it is important to ensure the integrity of all ventilator connections. The most frequent site of accidental disconnection from the ventilator is at the tracheostomy tube.[41] The risk of disconnection can be reduced by careful observation and by securing the connection with twill tape, shoelaces, or other ties during activity. The connection should not be secured so tightly, however, that it creates discomfort or compromises the child's airway.

Several additional safety precautions are warranted when a child is mechanically ventilated (see box, "Selected Safety Precautions"). When the nurse or parent is introducing the interventionist to the child's ventilation system, the interventionist should carefully note locations where the ventilator tubing might accidentally disconnect during treatment sessions. The interventionist also should note that when humidity is added to the inspired air, it is not uncommon for water to accumulate in the tubing. To prevent accidental spillage of this water into the child's airway, the nurse, parent, or other trained individual should empty the tubing before the treatment session and at any other time water accumulates.

Most ventilators used in the home have numerous dials and switches that affect the respiratory rate and other important aspects of ventilation. Settings are determined individually and should not be adjusted except under a physician's order. If they are accidentally knocked, the nurse, parent, or other trained individual should be summoned quickly to check them. Ventilators are equipped with alarms to signal pressure or volume alterations and electrical failure. The sounding of an alarm may represent an emergency, and the nurse, parent, or other trained individual should be summoned immediately.

A tracheostomy provides airway access for long-term mechanical ventilation. A tracheostomy also may be used to ensure an adequate airway in an infant whose

Selected Safety Precautions for Mechanical Ventilation

Secure ventilator tubing at tracheostomy tube to reduce the risk of accidental disconnection during movement.

Exercise caution in repositioning to prevent accidental disconnection of ventilator tubing.

Observe tubing for water accumulation and ask parent or nurse to empty as needed.

Avoid knocking or otherwise altering ventilator settings.

Summon parents or nurse promptly if alarm sounds or other problems occur.

tracheal airway has narrowed as a result of numerous intubations for resuscitation or of other disorders.

A tracheostomy affects communication development. Several excellent resources address this topic.[42–45] A tracheostomy itself does not interfere with most therapy treatment interventions. The child may naturally hyperextend the neck to ensure an adequate airway. Extreme flexion of the neck and any activities that may occlude the tracheostomy tube should be avoided. If the tracheostomy tube is not covered by the ventilator or other tubing, the interventionist should be careful to prevent aspiration of dust and other particles when the child is prone and on the floor. Parents can be asked to provide either a tracheostomy humidifying filter (Fig 2), a piece of nylon stocking, or a bandanna to loosely cover the tracheostomy tube during therapy sessions.

The infant or young child with a tracheostomy may require assistance to clear secretions. If secretions bubble or are coughed out the tracheostomy tube, they can be wiped off with a clean gauze pad. Signs indicating that the nurse or parent should be summoned to suction the tracheostomy tube have been identified. The interventionist should be aware that crying will not be audible in a child with a tracheostomy; the child should be observed carefully for other signs of distress.

Humidity is important to maintain loose secretions in the child with a tracheostomy. If the child does not require ventilation, humidity can be maintained for short periods by the use of room humidifiers, the administration of several drops of saline, or the use of a tracheostomy humidifying filter.[23] If the child's breathing begins to sound dry or raspy, the interventionist should notify the parent or nurse as additional humidity may be necessary.

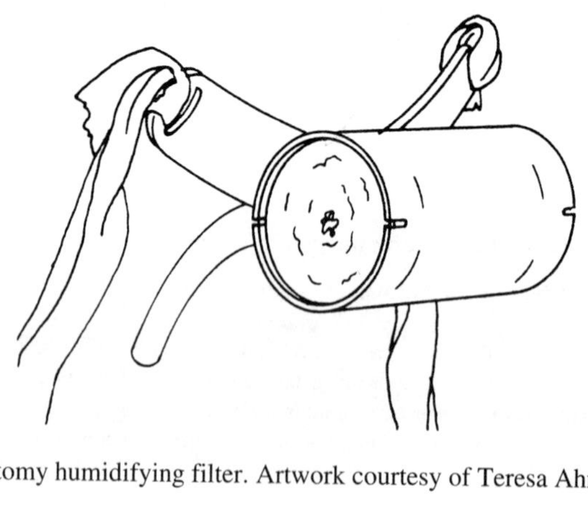

Fig 2. Tracheostomy humidifying filter. Artwork courtesy of Teresa Ahmann. © 1985.

Accidental decannulation of the tracheostomy tube is very rare, and the interventionist should not be unduly fearful about it. Should decannulation occur, it is an emergency, and the parent, nurse, or other trained individual should be summoned immediately to replace the tube. If services are not home based, program personnel should be trained in this emergency procedure.

Treatment program evaluation

Regular team meetings that include parents are important to coordinate and update service plans. The frequency of meetings should be based on several factors, including changes in the child's status, team design, and family preference.[12] The box, "Aspects of Evaluation," outlines important aspects of evaluation meetings.

Evaluation meetings ensure that programming ideas are shared and coordinated to promote gains in all areas of the child's development. For example, children with BPD often are at risk nutritionally and developmentally. For these children, expenditure of energy in a nonproductive, inefficient manner during therapy may limit growth. The net result may be a vicious cycle in which the child's tolerance for stimulation cannot be increased because he or she cannot gain or maintain weight, resulting in an energy deficit. As another example, the team can brainstorm about options for positioning the infant or providing greater mobility for the toddler. Evaluation meetings encourage professionals and families to work together to ensure that the developmental interventions contribute in a positive way to each child's overall progress.

• • •

Providing developmental intervention for the technology-dependent infant or young child is a challenging task that requires specialized medical, developmen-

Aspects of Evaluation of the Treatment Program

- statement of goals for child and family
- statement of measurable short- and long-term objectives
- documentation of actual treatment strategies
- documentation of actual progress on goals and objectives
- identification of factors interfering with treatment
- identification of differences in goals of various parties
- identification of possible conflicts in aspects of treatment
- assessment of communication between providers
- assessment of communication between providers and family
- revision of goals, objectives, treatment strategies, and communication plans
- documentation of revisions in treatment program

tal, and adaptive knowledge. A holistic approach should be taken that is sensitive to the child's medical, social, and developmental needs and to the family's needs and concerns. Intervention strategies must be flexible to accommodate changes in the child's status and the family's needs. Coordination of efforts among the various agencies and disciplines involved, accompanied by regular evaluation of goals, objectives, and strategies, will help ensure optimal gains in the child's medical and developmental status.

REFERENCES

1. US Congress, Office of Technology Assessment. *Technology-Dependent Children: Hospital v Home Care—A Technical Memorandum.* Washington, DC: Government Printing Office; 1987. Publication no. OTA-TM-H-38.
2. Johnson BH. Cited by: Kelly JF, Barnard KE. Early intervention. In: Wallace HM, Ryan G, Oglesby AC, eds. *Maternal and Child Health Practices.* 3rd ed. Oakland, Calif: Third Party Publishing; 1988.
3. Hanft B. The changing environment of early intervention services: Implications for practice. *Am J Occup Ther.* 1988;42:724–731.
4. Field T, Dempsey J, Shuman H. Developmental follow-up of pre- and post-term infants. In: Friedman SL, Sigman M, eds. *Preterm Birth and Psychological Development.* New York, NY: Academic Press; 1981.
5. Hunt I. Predicting intellectual disorders in childhood for preterm infants with birthweights below 1501 grams. In: Friedman SL, Sigman M, eds. *Preterm Birth and Psychological Development.* New York, NY: Academic Press; 1981.
6. Anderson J, Auster-Liebhaber J. Developmental therapy in the neonatal intensive care unit. *Phys Occup Ther Pediatr.* 1984;4:89–106.
7. Thomas R. A foundation for clinical family assessment. *Child Health Care.* 1990;19:244–250.
8. Wegener DH, Aday LA. Home care for ventilator-assisted children: Predicting family stress. *Pediatr Nurs.* 1989;15:371–376.
9. Ahmann E. *Home Apnea Monitoring and Patterns of Family Life.* Baltimore, Md: The Johns Hopkins University School of Hygiene and Public Health; 1989. Dissertation.
10. Thomas RB. *Ventilator Dependency Consequences for Child and Family.* Seattle, Wash: University of Washington School of Nursing; 1986. Dissertation.
11. Dalton R, Kirkhart K. An evolution of emotional problems faced by ventilator-assisted children. *Psych Forum.* 1985–86;13:73–81.
12. Turnbull A, Turnbull H. *Families, Professionals, and Exceptionalities: A Special Partnership.* Columbus, Ohio: Charles Merrill; 1986.
13. Consolvo C, Wade JE. Producing videos for home use by parents of high-risk infants. *Am J Maternal Child Nurs.* 1990;15:178–179.
14. Shelton T, Jeppson E, Johnson B. *Family Centered Care for Children with Special Health Care Needs.* Washington, DC: Association for the Care of Children's Health; 1987.
15. Johnson B, McGonigel M, Kaufmann R, eds. *Guidelines and Recommended Practices for the Individualized Family Service Plan.* Washington, DC: Association for the Care of Children's Health; 1989.

16. Thomas RB. Family adaptation to the child with a chronic condition. In: Rose MH, Thomas RB, eds. *Children with Chronic Conditions: Nursing in a Family and Community Context.* Orlando, Fla: Grune & Stratton; 1987.
17. Project Copernicus. *Recognizing Family-Centered Care: A Group Exercise.* Baltimore, Md: Kennedy Institute; 1990.
18. American Association of University Affiliated Programs. *Developing a Community Team.* Washington, DC: US Dept of Health and Human Services; 1982.
19. Haynes UB. The national collaborative infant project. In: Tjossem TD, ed. *Intervention Strategies for High Risk Infants and Young Children.* Baltimore, Md: University Park Press; 1976.
20. Woodruff G, McGonigel MG. Early intervention team models: The transdisciplinary approach. In: Gallagher J, Hutinger P, Jordan J, Karnes M, eds. *Early Childhood Special Education: Birth to Three.* Reston, Va: Council for Exceptional Children; 1988.
21. Bozynski MEA. Comprehensive management of the infant with bronchopulmonary dysplasia: A growing challenge. *Inf Young Children.* 1989;2:14–24.
22. Markestad T, Fitzhardinge PM. Growth and development in children recovering from bronchopulmonary dysplasia. *J Pediatr.* 1981;98:597–602.
23. Ahmann E. *Home Care for the High Risk Infant: A Holistic Guide to Using Technology.* Rockville, Md: Aspen; 1986.
24. Vohr BR, Bell EF, Oh W. Infants with bronchopulmonary dysplasia: Growth patterns and neurologic and developmental outcome. *Am J Dis Child.* 1982;136:443–447.
25. Whaley LF, Wong DL. The high risk newborn and family. In: Whaley LF, Wong DL, eds. *Nursing Care of Infants and Young Children.* St. Louis: C.V. Mosby; 1987.
26. Bancalari E, Gerhardt T. Bronchopulmonary dysplasia. *Pediatr Clin North Am.* 1988;33:1–23.
27. Goldson E. Severe bronchopulmonary dysplasia in the very low birthweight infant: Its relationship to developmental outcome. *J Dev Behav Pediatr.* 1984;5:165–168.
28. Als H, Lawhorn G, Brown E, et al. Individualized behavioral and environmental care for the very low birth weight preterm infant at high risk for bronchopulmonary dysplasia: Neonatal intensive care unit and developmental outcome. *Pediatrics.* 1986;78:1123–1132.
29. Anderson J. Sensory intervention with the preterm infant in the neonatal intensive care unit. *Am J Occup Ther.* 1986;40:19–26.
30. Boynton BR, Jones B. Nursing care of the infant with bronchopulmonary dysplasia. In: Ballard RA, ed. *Bronchopulmonary Dysplasia.* Boston, Mass: Blackwell Scientific; 1988.
31. Als H. Toward a synactive theory of development: Promise for the assessment and support of infant individuality. *Inf Ment Health J.* 1982;3:229–243.
32. Haynie M, Porter SM, Palfrey JS. *Children Assisted by Medical Technology in Educational Settings: Guidelines for Care.* Boston, Mass: The Children's Hospital, Project School Care; 1989.
33. Sherman LP, Rosen CD. Development of a preschool program for tracheostomy dependent children. *Pediatr Nurs.* 1990;16:357–361.
34. Hennessy P. *Home Care of Your Child With a Tracheostomy: A Parent Handbook.* Washington, DC: Children's Hospital National Medical Center; 1983.
35. Frates RC, Splaingard ML, Smith EO, et al. Outcomes of home mechanical ventilation in children. *J Pediatr.* 1985;106:850–856.
36. Katcher ML, Shapiro MM, Guist C. Severe injury and death associated with home infant cardiorespiratory monitors. *Pediatrics.* 1986;78:775–779.

37. Jennings C. An alternative: Nasal cannula oxygen therapy for infants who are oxygen dependent. *Am J Maternal Child Nurs.* 1982;7:89,92.

38. Voyles JB. Bronchopulmonary dysplasia. *Am J Nurs.* 1981;81:510–514.

39. Ellmyer P, Thomas NJ. A guide to your patient's safe home use of oxygen. *Nurs 82.* 1982;12:56–57.

40. Dougherty JM. Negative pressure devices in pediatric practice. *Pediatr Nurs.* 1990;16:135–138.

41. Janowski MJ. Accidental disconnections from breathing systems. *Am J Nurs.* 1984;84:241–243.

42. Simon BM, Fowler SM, Handler SD. Communication development in young children with long-term tracheostomies: Preliminary report. *Int J Pediatr Otorhinolaryngol.* 1983;6:37–50.

43. Kaslon KW, Grabo DE, Ruben R. Voice, speech and language habilitation in young children without laryngeal function. *Arch Otolaryngol.* 1978;104:737.

44. Simon B, Handler SD. The speech pathologist and management of children with tracheostomies. *J Otolaryngol.* 1981;19:440.

45. Simon BM. Speech and language development in the high risk infant. In: Ahmann E, ed. *Home Care for the High Risk Infant: A Holistic Guide to Using Technology.* Rockville, Md: Aspen; 1986.

Contingency, means-end skills, and the use of technology in infant intervention

Margaret W. Sullivan, PhD
Associate Professor of Pediatrics

Michael Lewis, PhD
Professor of Pediatrics and Psychiatry
Institute for the Study of Child Development
Development of Pediatrics
University of Medicine and Dentistry of New Jersey
Robert Wood Johnson Medical School
New Brunswick, New Jersey

IN THE LAST decade, technology, including simple switches for battery-operated toys and more sophisticated applications (such as computers with adapted access), has become available to professionals working with disabled and developmentally delayed children. Switches are any device that requires only simple or gross movement to deliver power. *Switch-adapted toys* and *switch-toy* technology are terms used in this article to describe any method by which battery-operated toys or other stimulus devices (such as tape recorders) are made readily accessible to the physically limited child by switches. Since Public Law 99-457 mandated services for the disabled preschool child, there has been particular interest in the use of technology for the preschooler with disabilities in both educational and play settings. Somewhat less attention has been devoted to the use of technology in infant intervention, particularly with infants younger than 1 year. A recent review notes that data on this age group are scarce.[1] In this article, we argue that switch-toy technology not only is developmentally appropriate for use in infant intervention but can also be appropriately introduced at developmental levels from 2 to 12 months. Finally, we offer some suggestions for integrating switch-adapted toys successfully and meaningfully into a learning curriculum for infants and children with disabilities with developmental functioning under 1 year of age.

CONTINGENCY, CONTROL, AND THE LEARNED HELPLESSNESS MODEL

To understand the theoretical importance of switch-adapted toys in early intervention, consider the concept of contingency as it is used in the infant learning literature. Contingency refers to a perceived relationship of either correlation or causality between two events. A contingency can exist between two stimuli or events, so that one serves as a signal or cue of the other. For example, if one

The data presented in this article are from a study funded by Robert Wood Johnson Foundation grant 10170. Preparation of this manuscript was supported by grant MCJ-110584 from the Maternal and Child Health Bureau (Title V, Social Security Act), Health Resources and Services Administration, Department of Health and Human Services. We gratefully acknowledge Richard P. Brinker, who developed the initial version of the curriculum and who first introduced Margaret W. Sullivan to this area.

Inf Young Children 1993; 5(4): 58–77

consistently pairs a number of tongue clicks with the insertion of a pacifier into a young infant's mouth, soon the tongue clicks alone will elicit mouth opening. Contingencies also often exist between one's own actions and the responses or outcomes that they produce. These outcomes may be social or physical events. For example, when an infant vocalizes and smiles, the mother vocalizes back. Soon the infant seems to initiate conversations. Both these examples are instances of conditioning (the first is classic conditioning, and the second is instrumental conditioning), but we and others in the field of infant development prefer the term *contingency learning* for these examples to emphasize the relation between meaningful events in the environment and the infant's active role in perceiving, controlling, and exploring them. The term *conditioning* implies that the control is external: The stimulus controls the behavior. Although this appears to be so in the case of laboratory animals and perhaps in the case of infants from the perspective of the experimenter, the subjects themselves may have another view of the matter.

Response-outcome contingencies are commonly mastered by young infants as motor development proceeds, as they swat, kick, bang, and otherwise manipulate objects encountered in their environment. We define contingency learning broadly as the process of becoming aware of such response-outcome relations and actively controlling or exploring them. Contingent events in the environment provide opportunities for infants actively to experience effective means for engaging the physical world and experiencing success at doing so. That which is contingent upon one's own behavior can be predicted, controlled, or exploited in a number of ways.

From the foregoing discussion, it is apparent that infants with motor and/or sensory deficits or delays (hereafter we use the term *disabled* to refer to these conditions) are at a disadvantage in learning action-outcome contingencies, particularly with objects. Consider the following two infants: Josh, a 3-month-old, is lying on his stomach and moving his hands along the sheets of the crib. His hand makes contact with a rattle. While he is continuing to move his hand, the rattle, which he is now touching quite by accident, makes a noise. Josh attends to the noise and attempts to grasp the rattle. He does not succeed, but it makes a noise again. This time, Josh smiles. He attempts to grasp the rattle again. Anthony is a 6-month-old, born 2 months prematurely, who experienced an intraventricular hemorrhage and subsequent brain damage. He has high spasticity in all extremities and does not move his arms or legs frequently. When he does, the movement is obligatory extension. Anthony rarely makes contact with the many available objects in his crib.

Given Anthony's motor capabilities, he has a much reduced probability of experiencing co-occurrences between his self-generated activity and environmental consequences compared with Josh. Even when Anthony accidentally encounters an interesting outcome contingent on his behavior, he will have great difficulty in effecting the movement to reproduce it. Therefore, Anthony cannot readily play with and explore objects; there is a deficit of action-outcome contingencies in Anthony's life.

It was the recognition of such a deficit that first led to a discussion of learned helplessness with respect to the disabled infant and how technology might serve to remedy poor motor functioning, thereby enhancing performance and presumably motivation.[2–6] Briefly, the learned helplessness model of motivation states that prolonged exposure to uncontrollable environmental events leads to withdrawal and passivity.[7] Experiences with an uncontrollable environment produce a generalized expectancy that the environment cannot be mastered and that it is not worth trying to do so. The child is primed to give up easily, does not try alternatives, or, in the extreme case, does not attempt to engage the environment at all. The model, derived originally from laboratory studies of avoidance conditioning in animals, has led to clinical applications in humans.[8–10] From the learned helplessness perspective, the purpose of switch-adapted toys is to allow the disabled infant and child opportunities of control. Learned helplessness can thus be prevented, and instead a generalized expectancy of control will be established. Such generalized expectancies of control are thought to be the roots of feelings of efficacy and mastery motivation.[11,12]

Often discussions of technology for the young disabled child focus almost exclusively on its role as first aid for learned helplessness. Although switch-toy technology and simple cause-effect computer games allow disabled children the opportunity to experience the powerful motivating effects of control, we have been dissatisfied with the learned helplessness model as the sole rationale and model for using technology, particularly in infant intervention. Learned helplessness describes only part of the impact that contingent events (or the lack of them) have on the young child. This motivational construct is basically a model of behavioral pathology or deficit (ie, it explains why motivation is lacking), yet it fails to inform the practitioner about how and when contingent activities will maximally inhibit or prevent learned helplessness.

Learned helplessness is a behavioral diagnosis without adequately specified prevention methods. In particular, because learned helplessness is not a developmental model, issues of how the infant's or child's developing cognitive capacities may contribute to stimulus preferences in the events that infants and children might enjoy controlling, or how effectively to foster a *generalized* notion of environmental control, are not addressed. Yet, after all, such information is what one is ultimately seeking in the attempt to stave off learned helplessness. For the educator or therapist who is attempting to develop practical applications with the young child, such a developmental model is needed. Information about when and how to begin to foster contingency learning through the use of switch-adapted toy technology is critical. Without it, poor or ineffective efforts are likely.

Finally, in the translation from the psychologic to the education literature, the message that learned helplessness develops rapidly and can be resistant to change has been underemphasized or lost. These two facts about learned helplessness alone suggest that efforts to prevent it should begin as early as possible and should be applied continuously and consistently in the child's therapeutic and educational programming and in daily life.

Although the learned helplessness model does not go far enough for the practitioner, two complementary sources familiar to all early childhood professionals provide considerable information for constructing a technology-based curriculum for environmental control. These two sources are Piagetian models of the development of means-end skills and infant contingency learning research. Both provide a strong rationale for introducing switch-toy technology in infancy. The infant learning literature in particular provides a wealth of practical information about how to construct a contingency curriculum that will foster generalized expectancies of control. After discussing each source, we present an outline of such a curriculum for young disabled infants that we have field tested.

MEANS-END SKILLS AND THE DEVELOPMENT OF EXPECTANCIES OF CONTROL

Piaget's[13] theory of sensorimotor development is a model for the infant's early intellectual or cognitive development. It describes how, over the course of the first 18 to 24 months of life, the infant develops, in stagelike steps, a number of basic concepts such as object permanence, means-end skills, and primitive action-based object classification (schemes). Piaget's model has gained wide acceptance as a general model of infant cognitive development, and two aspects of the model, the development of problem-solving skills and the development of schemes, directly bear on the infant's learning of control. For Piaget and other theorists, the infant's use of its own responses as means or tools for engaging the external environment and exploiting interesting events emerges in an invariant sequence from about the second month of life. The following discussion focuses on the opening months of life because our goal is to examine the development of learned expectancies of control.

Infants first become aware of responses as a means of controlling interesting events through what Piaget[13] termed circular reactions. These actions are circular because they are readily repeated by infants to reinstate any event that is first encountered accidentally. Initial occurrence appears to elicit recurrence, perhaps for pleasure or self-stimulation. Originally centered around stimuli and events related to the infant's own bodily activities such as hand-to-mouth movement, gross movements of the body, and sucking, circular reactions become increasingly directed toward objects and events in the wider environment after about the third or fourth month. Now termed secondary circular reactions, the infant's responses are fairly discrete, specific behaviors clearly directed toward specific objects and persons in the environment. These secondary circular reactions, describe by Piaget,[13] are semi-intentional; that is, the infant did not purposefully set out to cause the outcome (although it perceived the response-outcome relation once it occurred) but purposefully attempted to reproduce the relation.

Piaget[13] observed that circular reactions are repeated with much enjoyment by infants in a playful manner, first with familiar objects and subsequently with novel objects. Indeed, he supposed that joy constantly springing up helps maintain their circular nature. Subsequently, these well-practiced reactions become the basis of the infant's relating to and exploring objects during play. Data available on the development of schemes from the Uzgiris-Hunt Scales of Infant Ordinal Development,[14] an assessment tool based on Piaget's model, indicate that by 5 to 6 months most infants will systematically use several secondary circular reactions in playful explorations of objects. These early and simple aspects of discovering action-outcome relations and their repetition and exploitation during play are recognized as fundamental to early cognitive development. The only point of disagreement between Piagetian and other recent models of infant cognitive development[15] seems to be whether primary and later circular reactions are separate stages.

Our choice of terminology and discussion should make clear that we regard circular reactions and action-outcome contingencies as one and the same. Even schemes can be understood as contingencies that have been overgeneralized and have become methods for exploring objects. An infant who has had sufficient experience with shaking a multitude of objects to obtain interesting sounds will come to have a generalized expectation that shaking objects yields interesting effects and will use this generalized response in play with novel objects. The infant will first apply this scheme to those objects encountered that are most similar to rattles. By and by, the infant will apply this scheme in exploring any novel object. Thus, assessment of schemes should provide a good index of the degree to which experience with object contingencies has yielded generalized expectations about how objects can be exploited.

IMPLICATIONS OF COGNITIVE-DEVELOPMENTAL MODELS FOR A MEANS-END CURRICULUM

The heart of the message that Piagetian models have for a technology curriculum is that the ability to use one's responses as tools (means) to obtain a desired goal (end) in the environment does not miraculously emerge full-blown at 12 or even at 18 months. Flexible, playful, insightful use of means-end skills is a problem-solving technique originating in early, simple experiences of environmental contingency. In the earliest months, these experiences require little in the way of coordinated motor behavior. Only gross actions on the part of the infant are necessary. Motor actions must be correlated or contiguous with interesting events or some positive change in the infant's immediate environment, and these events must occur consistently. For disabled infants, this implies that it is imperative to begin providing contingent experiences in the physical environment as soon as the motor deficit is suspected. Technology can function as a prosthetic device to mimic the earliest experiences of secondary circular reactions.[6]

A second implication is that the initial contingency experiences of the infant, and indeed all the experiences that drive means-end problem-solving skills, are self-discovered. As such, they are the infant's first experiences of its own agency and are powerfully motivating. The infant will not need to be nagged or prompted to control a particular stimulus event provided that the event is interesting and in the infant's control. Recognition of the event's relation to self-action will lead naturally to sufficient repetitions until the event no longer holds interest or, as Piaget would have said, until it has been assimilated. This repetition is particularly important because, even at the earliest stages of control, Piaget[13] believed that repetitions were intentional although the original act was not.

From this, we can draw two conclusions. First, it is necessary to arrange the environment (or to position the child within it) so that the child has both a high probability of discovering control of the interesting event by chance and a high probability of repeating the movement that accidentally leads to contingency. The environment in a means-end program is defined as the sum total of all the technology and adapted devices needed to allow the child easily to make and repeat a response or a set of responses and to detect the occurrence of stimulus events. In other words, the environment is the switches, how they are mounted, how the child is supported, and where the contingent event is staged for easy and comfortable attention. Second, the event must be something that is of interest to the child. It is not difficult to find events that interest children, but battery-adapted toys and other electronically produced events must be suited to the child's sensory preferences. They must be neither too loud nor too soft. The developmental aspects of the toy must also be taken into account. A drumming, whistling monkey dressed as an Indian Chief or a singing purple octopus with red flashing eyes (both of which were sold as adapted toys) will delight a young infant who enjoys color and sound and the facelike quality of both these toys. The older infant, however, will find them bizarre and quite possibly frightening. Even given the most appropriate and enjoyable contingency event, the infant is likely to lose interest with time, so that availability of different novel contingency outcomes is desirable. Novel toys sustain interest and promote response repetition, thereby consolidating the scheme.

The final implication to be drawn from this discussion is related to cognitive growth and generalization. Circular reactions ultimately become generalized schemes for exploring and manipulating objects during play. They will be used to explore novel objects and events and will ultimately be combined to yield new, coordinated activities on objects. Therefore, an effective means-end curriculum must use switches within and across contexts and with various familiar and novel toys.

LESSONS FROM THE CONTINGENCY LITERATURE

These fairly specific recommendations for a means-end curriculum provide us with a general working outline of an adapted toy program for infants that is based on a cognitive-developmental perspective. This perspective also dictates when and why contingency experiences should be introduced to foster cognition: as early as possible in infancy. The infant contingency learning literature also indicates the specific behavioral effects of an infant's experiences of contingency.

At least three distinct effects of contingencies have been discussed prominently in the developmental literature. First, contingencies affect attention. They alert and orient the infant to the physical environment and serve to modulate or maintain attention.[16] Second, the detection and mastery of contingencies lead to positive emotional behaviors such as smiling and vocalizing[17,18] and may suppress negative emotion.[19] Third, memory for contingencies becomes the impetus for subsequent intentional actions and, ultimately, for the development of expectancies and other cognitive structures. Those who act and remember how to react develop cognitively. The evidence that contingencies are facilitative of infant motivational, attentional, and cognitive development derives from both laboratory studies and studies of naturally occurring social contingencies (ie, mothers' responsivity to their infants).

Attention

Contingencies are clearly attention getting. Rovee-Collier and Fagen[20] and Sullivan et al[21] reported asymptotic levels of attention over 9 minutes of acquisition in the mobile paradigm, a remarkable attention span given 3-month-old subjects. Attention in these studies was defined as gaze oriented upward toward a multicolored mobile. Attention to contingent events has also been studied as the particular facial configuration of interest.[18] The facial expression of interest gives a more conservative estimate of the infant's active attention to the contingent stimulus because a simple fixation measure may obscure qualitative differences in infant attention. The fixated stimulus may be interesting, surprising, or fear producing. The results show that infants not only fixate on the contingent stimulus but also show interest, excitement, and surprise.

Differences between interest levels of infants receiving contingent as opposed to noncontingent presentations of a given stimulus occur over the course of exposure to the contingent event.[22] Although some types of noncontingent stimuli may elicit substantial amounts of attention in an alert infant,[23] attention to noncontingent stimuli is also likely to habituate (indeed, this is the basis of an entire literature on early infant information processing). If the noncontingent stimuli are unpredictable, infant fussing or crying will occur.[24] In either case, infants will not persist in attending to noncontingent events, although initial interest levels may not differ.[16]

Related to this discussion is a second aspect of the relation of contingencies to attention: Contingent stimulation appears to sustain longer periods of active interest and is related to better subsequent habituation. These effects have been observed both in life and in the laboratory. In a study of 3-month-olds, Lewis and Goldberg[25] compared overall maternal stimulation (as measured by the frequency of the mother's talking to, smiling at, or holding the infant) to the contingent responsivity of the mother (as measured by how much she engaged in these behaviors after her infant vocalized and smiled). Two classes of maternal behavior, overall stimulation level and contingent responsivity, were found to be related differentially to infant ability to habituate to a redundant signal and to attend to a novel one. Such habituation/novelty tasks are early measures of attention or information processing. Contingent maternal responsivity was found to be more related to these measures of infant information processing than total amount of maternal stimulation. Maternal responsivity rather than maternal stimulation (either proximal or distal stimulation) was found to be significantly related to 3-month-olds' concurrent scores on the Bayley Scales of Infant Mental Development.[26] Likewise, Lewis and Freedle[27] reported that the mother's contingent vocalization was related to the infant's subsequent language development.

Recent laboratory replication of the effects of prior contingent and noncontingent social stimulation on the concurrent information processing of infants was described by Dunham and colleagues.[28,29] They reported that prior contingent stimulation was associated with better habituation performance immediately after the contingent exposure and that contingent vocal engagement during interaction was associated with better subsequent performance on a nonsocial contingency task. In other words, contingency learning, defined as responsivity of the infants' environment, enhanced both habituation and subsequent social interaction.

Because the evidence from several of the above studies is correlational, it is impossible to determine whether maternal responsivity caused improved attention and cognitive functioning or whether precocious infants elicited more maternal responsivity.[30] Nevertheless, the data demonstrate that maternal responsivity exerts its effects on infant development early in the infant's life and involves touching, looking, and smiling.

Lewis et al[16] studied infants 10, 16, and 24 weeks of age in the laboratory and found support for a causal link between environmental contingency and motivation. Half the infants in each age group were experimental subjects, and half were control subjects. Both groups were seated in a test booth before a rear-projection screen. For the experimental group, a string was attached to the infant's wrist so that a slight pull would result in a 3-second presentation of a colored slide accompanied by children's voices singing. Thus the experimental group's action (pulling) produced a contingent outcome. Each control subject received the same amount of stimulation as a matched experimental subject of the same age and sex. The programmed stimulation was generated for control subjects by playing back a recording of the matched (yoked) experimental subject's performance.

Subjects who received contingent stimulation differed from those who received noncontingent stimulation in three ways: They learned to pull the string to turn on the picture, they remained in the experimental setting longer before becoming fussy and crying, and they smiled more as a consequence of the contingency between their behavior and picture onset. Contingent subjects remained alert and interested in the procedure for an average of 17 minutes, and the noncontingent subjects stayed interested and did not fuss for only 8 minutes. Moreover, these differences between contingent and noncontingent subjects occurred at all ages. They emerged in spite of the fact that there were no differences in the frequency of stimulation for the groups. Contingent stimulation served to maintain attention and arousal better than noncontingent stimulation.

Emotional consequences

Contingency experience is enjoyable to even the youngest infants. The laboratory results described above documented this fact, corroborating and extending the anecdotal reports and data of others.[17,18,21] Subsequent work on cognition and emotion has expanded upon these original findings.[19,22,31] Specifically, facial expressions of interest and enjoyment increase when infants control contingent events in the environment, and matched-to-level noncontingent events produce little positive emotion or engagement and lead to early fussing and withdrawal. Conversely, infants who receive contingent stimulation show little negative emotion, suggesting that contingent stimulation may suppress negative arousal. Negative emotion occurs in response to deprivation. When given contingent experience and then deprived of it, infants at even the youngest ages (10 weeks) will increase the specific activity associated with control of the consequence (pulling) and will show anger at the unexpected loss of control.[22,32]

Gekoski and colleagues,[33] in a study of latency to quiet and renewal of crying upon cessation of maternal soothing, reported that some infants began developing expectancies about the social consequences of caretaker behavior as early as 6 weeks of age. Over the course of several months, latency to quiet decreased dramatically in all subjects, and anticipatory quieting to the approach of the soother was observed in some infants. Thus infants learned to modulate their negative state in response to contingent/maternal intervention.

From these studies it can be concluded that increased positive emotion and decreased negative emotion occur even with brief exposure to contingent stimulation. This effect is likely to be enhanced over time when the contingency experience is repeated. Sullivan and colleagues[21] reported, for example, that smiling in response to a mobile contingency tended to increase over days of exposure. The link between emotion and contingency may serve as the basis of infants' emerging motivational systems. The laboratory studies of contingency also demonstrate that environmental consequences need not be social in nature to be effective in promoting these effects, nor does the motor response need to be particularly well coordinated. This last fact is particularly important to the infant with motor disabilities. In our laboratory,[20] infants who have not learned to reach readily master nonsocial contingencies between arm movements and objects. There is little difference in learning between infants with and without Down syndrome as long as infants with Down syndrome are well supported physically.[34]

Contingency, expectancy, and generalization

The last effect of contingencies on the child is the formation of expectancies regarding the relations of self-generated responses. Although the notion of expectancies has been discussed in psychology for some time, there has been little discussion of how such expectancies with regard to environmental control might develop and generalize in young infants. In part, there has been a reluctance to acknowledge the role of memory in the contingency learning of young infants, yet having an expectancy of control implies that one remembers something about a stimulus, a response, or the relation between them. This is an extremely conservative position. The study of memory for contingent events has revealed remarkable infant abilities and suggests that memory for specific contingency events is a salient aspect of early cognitive development.

Rovee-Collier and Fagen[20] have demonstrated that infants are capable of more than basic recognition memory. Infants 2 to 3 months of age are capable of cued recall. That is, infants will produce the appropriate previously learned response when a formerly contingent stimulus is presented to them as a cue. Infants communicate to the experimenter that they remember the stimulus by producing the motor action. In the protocol developed by Rovee-Collier and Fagen,[20] infants readily learned a contingency between their foot kicks and movement of an overhead mobile. Infants at this age often dramatically increased kicking over 9 minutes of training on each of 2 days. Twenty-four hours later, the presence of the nonmoving mobile over the crib triggered foot kicking at a level similar to the final training level attained previously by the infant.[35] Infants not only recognized the formerly contingent stimulus but remembered that its occurrence was associated with a particular response. Infants remembered what to do to control the mobile. This memory is the basis of an expectancy of control. It is an expectancy about a specific response and a specific contingent outcome.

In more than 10 years of research on various aspects of infant memory for contingent mobiles, a number of findings have emerged that show that a more generalized expectancy of control may become established. The results are drawn almost exclusively from the work of Rovee-Collier and Fagen[20] on the mobile contingency, but there is no reason to suppose that the data are not generalizable to other contingency contexts. Briefly, memory for contingencies is excellent, given even short training, and can persist for as long as 2 weeks.[20,21,36] Memory for the contingent consequence is quite specific. Substitution of a novel mobile for the original training one disrupts retention for an interval of 4 days after training, suggesting that novelty is recognized.[35,37] Not just any mobile hung over the crib will elicit kicking after training.[38] After the 4-day interval, however, infants tend to respond to the general class of mobiles with kicking. Even after the original memory of the contingency itself has apparently been forgotten (2 weeks or even 1 month after training), infants can be reminded by reexposure to the contingent consequence.[39,40] As long as the reminding event includes the specific stimulus with which the infant was trained,[41] infants exposed to a reactivation will kick, whereas those whose memories have not been so primed will not.

Infants will generalize to a class of contingent events if they are exposed to various exemplars during training.[42] In another study, providing infants with a different mobile on each of three training days allowed infants to generalize readily to a novel mobile on a fourth (test) day. Instead of the inhibition typically seen in response to a novel mobile, the infants came to expect novelty and kicked as though they expected any mobile to be played with in this fashion.

The context in which the contingency occurs is a critical part of the event at the earliest ages.[41,43] Changes in context (a different crib liner or a different room) can inhibit memory of the contingency, but the detrimental effects of contextual change on contingency memory can be alleviated by providing common contingency experiences in multiple settings.[44]

This remarkable set of findings offers an outline of how generalized expectancies of control develop as the infant initiates even gross motor exploration, perhaps even before the onset of directed reaching. Starting sometime between the first and second month, the infant becomes aware of contingencies between its motor behavior and events in the environment. Exactly when this occurs is variable, depending in part on the infant's neurophysiologic maturity, but it has already occurred by early in the second month. This awareness requires a certain level of alertness and ability to attend to events but only a fairly gross level of motor ability. Activity level may also be a factor in that more active infants will be more likely accidentally to discover contingencies. Likewise, their early discovery and manipulation of contingencies will be more obvious to parents.[45] Parents, presumably delighted by the infant's play, may be more motivated to arrange circumstances for systematic future occurrences (ie, practice) leading to the perfecting of the particular responses. Even infants with low activity levels, however, if given enough time to discover an interesting contingent event and a response that is not too energy intensive, will manipulate contingencies, although the level and the vigor of their response may be less than those of a more active child.

To call these early contingency learning experiences simple conditioned behavior is misleading. From the outset, there has been some discrimination and other incidental learning on the part of the infant. For example, infants at 3 months of age learn in a small number of exposures to contingencies which one of four limbs controls the mobile and which three do not.[46] Likewise, the context-dependent nature of contingency memory implies that incidental learning occurs regarding salient characteristics of the total environment in which the contingency was encountered. This is highly adaptive because it means that there will be many features available to the alert infant that can trigger the infant's expectancy subsequently. The prototypic contingency memory is, therefore, episodic and highly context specific, and the infant's expectancy regarding its response and the contingent outcome is also quite specific, at least initially. Even fairly small variations in elements of a stimulus will disrupt infant performance, resulting in exploratory responses (attention and response testing).[47] These small variations in the contingent stimulus are mastered fairly rapidly by normal infants, however. Gross changes in the contingent stimulus will continue to disrupt infant response for several (about 4) days,[37] although this may vary with the salience of the particular change and the cognitive abilities of the child. After this interval the infant's memory of the original contingency event presumably has become sufficiently indistinct that any generally similar stimulus triggers the memory, and the infant will respond expectantly to it.

This 4-day limit on memory for specific details of the contingent stimulus appears to allow naturally for generalization to similar classes of stimuli. Some generalization of infant response occurs as the infant forgets specific details of the contingent stimulus while still remembering how to control objects of the same general class, resulting in a generalized expectancy about the probability of that response's controlling events. There is, however, at least one other way—training response to novelty[42]—that also leads to generalized expectancy. Experiencing contingencies with constantly novel outcomes seems to prime an infant to expect that novel events are controllable by the particular response.

Although the specificity of initial contingency memory suggests strict associations between responses and contingent outcomes, this does not seem to be the case, at least not for long. Normal infants by 6 months appear to hold independent expectancies about responses and contingent events.[48] They can spontaneously transfer prior knowledge of response to or control of outcome to new problems. There are no age changes in raw data on response rate or acquisition rate between 6 and 8 months.[49] It seems that generalized expectations about using one's responses to control the environment are in place by 6 to 8 months. Moreover, expectancy knowledge can be used flexibly and interchangeably to generate new contingency combinations.

Consider an infant's encounter with a rattle. When the rattle is grasped for the first time, the infant has no idea of the consequence. Accidentally, in the course of the infant's moving the hand holding the rattle, the rattle makes a sound. The infant will repeat this action many times with this specific rattle. Perhaps at first the infant will play with it in this fashion only in one position (eg, during diaper changes on the dressing table), the one in which it was originally encountered. The mother, however, may present the rattle to the infant in other positions and in other contexts. The infant will come to develop a generalized expectancy about shaking this rattle. If the infant is then provided with a similar rattle, the shaking contingency will generalize to it readily. The greater the variety of contexts in which the infant encounters them, the more the infant will come to expect that objects of a certain size, shape, and weight can be manipulated to produce auditory consequences. One might say that this is a concept of rattle or an action scheme of shaking. If the variety of objects that the infant has encountered as shakeable has been sufficiently large and occurs across a broad range of contexts, the shaking scheme will be so generalized that the infant will apply it even to novel objects. The infant will have acquired an expectancy about shaking and will attempt to explore and master novel objects by doing so, as suggested originally by Piaget.[13]

APPLICATIONS TO THE TECHNOLOGY CURRICULUM

What does this all mean for a teacher trying to develop a switch-toy curriculum? It means at least the following.

There is no ideal age or particular level of cognitive or motor skill required to begin

Any infant or child with a minimum developmental function of 2 to 3 months should be able to learn a simple contingency in some sensory modality. The response chosen can be a gross motor movement, as long as it is one that the child makes intermittently and is to some degree voluntary. A minimum level of alertness is necessary (it is also true that an appropriately chosen toy, when presented contingently, will enhance attention and interest[16] and so can be used to promote interest as a goal). A response that is not too fatiguing can be used to activate a switch independently for periods ranging from a minimum of 4 to 15 minutes. These minimum parameters have been confirmed in our contingency intervention work over the last 10 years with many infants and preschoolers with moderate, severe, and profound disabilities. More profoundly impaired children learn more slowly and require more creativity in positioning, switch selection, and mounting, but they do indeed learn.[4,50]

By way of illustration, Table 1 summarizes the contingency intervention histories of five infants who participated in a 3-month contingency intervention program.[51] Each received a contingency intervention system to use at home while enrolled in a standard early intervention program. The computer monitoring sys-

Table 1. Summary of intervention histories of infants who received contingency intervention

	Child				
Paramater	*TJ*	*Colin*	*Anthony*	*Zachary*	*Casey*
Age (weeks) at outset of program	24	34	34*	45*	45
Birth status	Full term	Full term	12 weeks premature	14 weeks premature	Full term
Known disabilities	Trisomy 21	Trisomy 21	Cerebral palsy, spastic	Cerebral palsy, spastic, some visual impairment	Microcephaly, cerebral palsy, spastic, hearing impairment, seizures
Program length (weeks)	12	10	13	14	13
Number of switches attempted	5	5	4	2	2
Number of toys experienced	10	11	12	8	9
Contingencies mastered	Arm Arm novel toy Arm toy change Leg Leg novel toy Leg toy change Leg arm shift Leg arm shift, novel toys Shift between novel switches Shift novel toys	Right arm RIght arm novel toy Right arm toy change Leg Leg novel toy Leg toy change Right arm leg shift Left arm Left arm novel toy Left arm leg shift Left arm right arm shift	Arm Arm novel toy Arm toy change Leg toy change Arm leg shift	Arm Arm novel toy Leg novel toy	Leg Leg novel toy

*Corrected for prematurity.

tem provided preprogrammed contingencies that were varied on a weekly basis. It also recorded infant data so that program changes could be made on the basis of evidence of mastery. Mothers provided the actual interventions over approximately a 3-month period and were requested to use the systems at least three times per week for up to 14 minutes at a time. These five children illustrate the range of physical and mental disabilities represented in the study and had mothers who complied with the minimum use requirements of the program. Table 1 shows that the children with the least disabling conditions mastered more contingencies, learned them in fewer sessions, and were able to respond appropriately to changes in the contingencies. The first three children, TJ, Colin, and Anthony, averaged one new toy weekly and mastered several different contingent responses alone and in combination. In contrast, Zachary learned two contingencies but more slowly relative to the others, and Casey, a child with multiple sensory and motor disabilities and frequent seizures, failed to master more than a single simple contingency. Nevertheless, Casey was able to use this contingency effectively to control a number of different toys. All these children were younger than 12 months.

It has been our experience in training classroom teachers and speech teachers that these professionals consistently underestimate the ability of severely impaired infants and children to use switches. This is the case despite reports of successful contingency learning in this population.[5,50,52] When asked to report on the minimum developmental age necessary for an infant to begin to benefit from such devices, most teachers report 6 to 9 months on preworkshop questionnaires. This mistaken attitude is reflected in teacher behavior. When children with whom to begin contingency training (switch-toy training) are selected, children with the poorest motor ability tend to be overlooked.

During training workshops, we have asked teachers to select three types of children for a contingency program: child A, who without doubt can learn to use switches; child B, who probably can learn but for whom the teacher envisions some difficulty; and child C, for whom learning is doubtful. Teachers have no problem making these designations, and the children they select tend to have similar characteristics by category. Child A is usually one who is already able to sit at a table or in an adapted chair with a tray and who is fairly visually alert. Child B also tends to be alert but has greater motor and attention or sensory problems. Usually, child B is quite spastic and does not tolerate sitting well, so that the repertoire of obvious physical movements with which to work is limited. Child C typically has the most profound motor involvement of the three. Multiple sensory deficits may be present. Usually this child cannot sit upright. Tone may be high or low, but apparently voluntary movements are infrequent, slight, or thought not to occur.

Teacher perceptions about children A and B are accurate; both children tend to master the initial contingency chosen. Invariably, teachers tend to be surprised by the performance of child C. It has been our experience that 75% of the time C children learn, sometimes within a single session. There seems to be a strong and natural bias on the part of teachers to provide switch-toy activities to those children (typically A children) in whom they have observed subtle evidence of already existing contingency behavior or who seem alert and ready for table activities. Children with poorer motor, postural, and attention skills who have not spontaneously shown evidence of means-end behavior, however, also can learn these activities. Ironically, they may be the very ones who may benefit most from contingency intervention and who need more intensive experience with contingencies to develop a generalized sense of control and the motive to move and explore. For these children, technology—the switches and the ability of the computer to track movement over time—does indeed serve as a behavioral microscope revealing latent learning capacity.[53]

The child must do it independently

To foster an expectation of control and to give the child the opportunity to learn to explore and discriminate among voluntary actions, it is critical that the response producing the contingency be self-initiated and performed independently. Shaping of responses initially (as in the traditional behavioral methods) is permissible but should be used sparingly. Shaping it may be necessary in cases where the child needs to learn which part of the switch is critical or where responses of only a certain strength will close the switch contacts. Shaping may also be necessary in the case of visually limited children in the initial stages of learning to orient them to the switch's location. Verbal prompting, verbal reinforcement, and hand-over-hand prompting of switch contact are not necessary if switches, positioning, and toys are appropriately selected. The environment itself must be so designed that the child's action is not excessively fatiguing and can be reliably reproduced. If the child is not successful, consider first restructuring the environment rather than resorting to prompting methods that effectively remove the child's possibility of choice and control.

Variety is the key to continued performance

It is absolutely critical to keep the contingent consequences interesting and meaningful for the child. No child will continue to control or manipulate a toy or event that is not enjoyable or interesting in some way. This means that toys and events must be varied, perhaps even within a play session when response and interest falter. No child, even one with limited attention span, can be expected to play continually with the same toy. To a large degree, the limited range of stimulation offered by battery-operated toys is a real problem (how different is a drumming bear from a drumming rabbit?), particularly if the child with severe or profound disability has more cognitive ability. One need not be limited to battery-operated mechanical toys, however. There are ways with even fairly simple technology to add sound to toys that have none and to switch-adapt standard electrical devices safely. Ultimately once means-end understanding has progressed sufficiently, switches can provide access to the computer itself. At this point, stimulus variety and value are greater.

Vary postures and contexts as much as possible once learning has occurred

This strategy promotes generalization or the functional use of a single specific response to new situations. The long-range goal is broader than to have the child play with any single toy or device. Ultimately, the goal is for the child to understand that a particular movement or response makes the world work.

Work with multiple responses if the child's repertoire permits

To promote a generalized expectancy of control, it is critical to work with more than one response from the outset. Infants may never begin their contingency experiences with a single response system. From birth, both sucking and head turning at least are available responses that can be used to explore contingent outcomes. Rapid physical development continuously expands this behavioral repertoire. Working with only a single switch fosters only an overlearned response to that switch. Furthermore, it deprives the child of an opportunity to discriminate among responses that are possible in an environment and stifles any innate tendency that may exist for the child to explore other movements spontaneously. Providing two switches simultaneously also allows ultimately for the introduction of solving a problem or making a choice. Therefore, it is important to have two possible responses or switches available from the outset and to introduce distinctive contingencies for each as soon as possible. When expectancy of control has generalized, the child understands and expects that there are multiple ways of controlling the environment and that some responses are appropriate some of the time but not all responses are appropriate all the time.

A WORKING CONTINGENCY CURRICULUM

To illustrate our recommendations as concretely as possible, we present in detail a contingency curriculum that was field tested in a recent study. The project was conducted over a 4-year period with 124 developmentally delayed infants from 4 to 15 months of age, all of whom were functioning at less than 12 months cognitively. Infants with Down syndrome and cerebral palsy represented the largest diagnostic groups, although infants with developmental delays of other and unknown etiologies were included in the sample. The study has been described in detail.[51] Briefly, each child received a computer at home for 3 months for contingency activities and automatic data recording. Progress throughout the program was monitored, and programming was changed weekly by a trained staff member. Changes in contingencies (switches and toys or both) were dependent on the infant's learning record. Although the computer, its software, and the mounting panel were custom designed for the project, the majority of switches, toys, and other adapted devices were purchased from commercial sources available to the professional community. Some toys purchased directly from store shelves were adapted by our technician. What we describe, then, is a program that can readily be replicated with existing, commercially available items and relatively low-cost technology. The computer, with its data collection system, display feature, and ability to modify programs flexibly, is not absolutely necessary, although it is desirable. Paper and pencil recording by an observer with a stopwatch or event recorder is equally satisfactory although more time consuming in terms of data analysis.

Goals

The contingency intervention had four goals, all of which were met for the majority of infants in the project: (1) to use the infant's self-initiated activity to enhance attention to physical events in the environment, (2) to teach the infant one or more means (responses or switches) for controlling interesting events in the immediate context, (3) to expose the infant to a number of controlling interesting events, and (4) to move systematically from mastery of simple contingent control to more complex contingency problems. All the above goals should serve to foster generalized attempts to control the environment and means-end understanding. We do not claim that the steps described are an invariant, or even the best, sequence for achieving such understanding. Rather, we offer them as a theoretically derived model that, as judged from our data, met the goals we set and to which disabled infants responded as we had predicted. All the figures illustrating the contingency concepts described below are from infants in the project. The figures were typically made in the home shortly after the session itself by the interventionist and were displayed for the parent.

Concept 1: Contingency awareness ("Something seems to happen when I move")

When an infant first encounters a contingent event, it is quite by accident, and the infant is unaware of the specific activity associated with the event. The contingency alerts the infant to the consequences of its own activity, however, and activity increases generally. This is a primary circular reaction described by Piaget.[13]

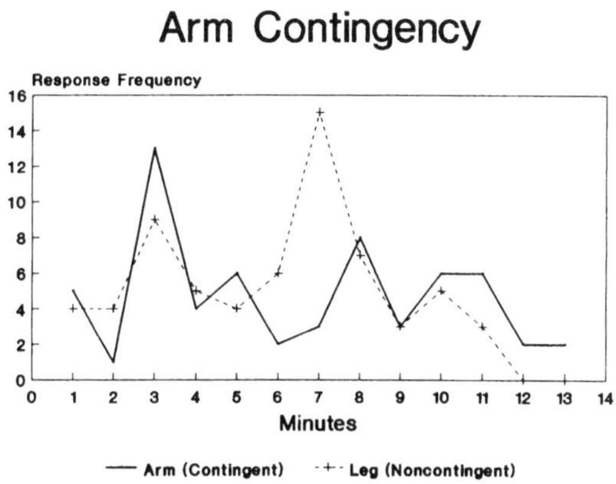

Fig 1. Contingency awareness in an infant with cerebral palsy.

Fig 1 provides an illustration of this response. Fig 1 shows both arm and leg responses over a 13-minute session in which a musical television toy served as the contingent outcome for a young infant with cerebral palsy. Although arm (the contingent) response was dominant at several points during the session, both arm and leg responses tended to increase over the course of the session. The infant had not isolated which response controlled the outcome. We have found that this type of response does not persist for long except in the most cognitively impaired infants. Many infants seem to identify the contingent response with a single session, despite significant motor disability.

Concept 2: Contingency learning ("This particular response makes something interesting happen")

The infant is aware that a specific response controls an interesting outcome. Although the contingency is accidentally discovered, subsequent repetitions are increasingly intentional, and it is clear that the infant understands that a relationship exists between action and outcome. This is a secondary circular reaction described by Piaget[13] and is illustrated in Fig 2. A drumming bear was the contingent outcome. The left arm response quickly became dominant. It is remarkable that the leg response dropped out almost entirely (conservatively, the noncontingent leg response should be emitted at random because it is being neither reinforced nor punished). The infant quickly became highly efficient and concentrated its activity on the response that paid off.

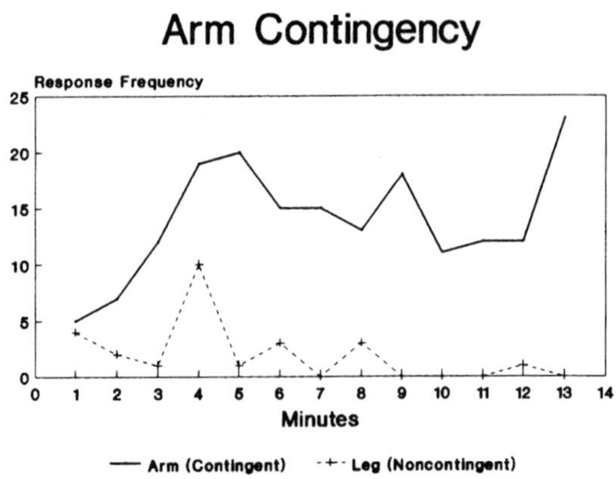

Fig 2. Learning of a left pulling contingency by a young infant with cerebral palsy.

Concept 3: Recovery of contingent response to novel consequences ("This response can make a variety of interesting things happen")

All contingencies, no matter how interesting, become boring with sufficient repetition. This is called habituation and is marked by a decline in attention and in the contingent response. The brighter the child, the duller the toy, and the more frequent the repetition, the more rapidly habituation will occur. In our work with nondisabled infants, we have found that the contingency will usually be mastered within 4 to 6 minutes, with interest declining thereafter. Although disabled infants may take longer initially to master the contingency, maximum play time with a contingent toy will fall within this same 4- to 6-minute window with familiarization. Thereafter, the contingent response will decline rapidly unless a novel toy is introduced. Introduction of a novel toy offers more than a method of overcoming habituation of a response, however. It also tests the infant's ability to generalize the response to a new outcome. Recovery of the contingent response is not automatically ensured, as is recovery of attention. The novel toy will indeed cause children to attend (they notice that something is different), but the contingent response may not rebound immediately. The child with poor generalization skills may be confused and revert to the level of primary circular reaction or may explore the noncontingent response as an option.

Fig 3 illustrates a good generalization response. An infant with Down syndrome initially learned to control a barking puppy with a leg response. Fig 3 shows that a familiar toy was responded to most vigorously in the first 2 minutes but that by 3 and 4 minutes responding had dropped off. The computer, programmed to monitor responses for signs of habituation, was instructed to make a new toy available for leg responses if the contingent response was below a response level typical for that

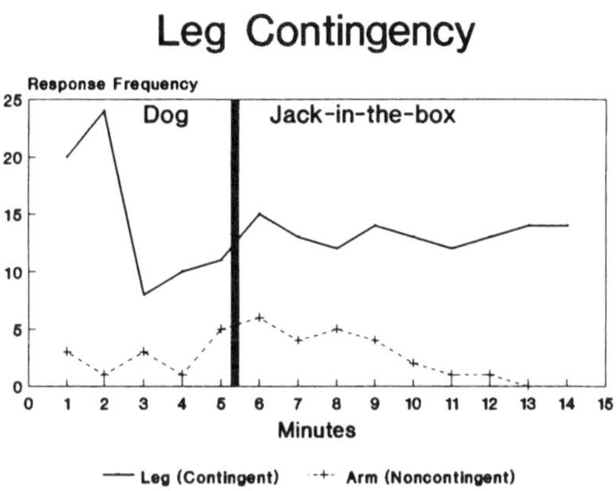

Fig 3. Recovery of leg responses by a young infant with Down syndrome with introduction of a toy change after 5 minutes of contingent play.

---

child (15 responses per minute) after 5 minutes. Fig 3 shows that the leg response did recover or generalize to the new toys and remained fairly stable through the end of the session. The lower rate of response to the new toy, in contrast to the familiar toy, is not unusual and may have resulted from either a cautious response to the novel event or a preference for the barking puppy, the familiar toy. In any case, what is critical is the recovery and maintenance of the correct response in the face of a change in the contingency problem.

Concept 4: Introduction of a new contingency ("Another response can make something happen")

It is important to provide the infant with strategies for exploring situations that have the potential for control even if the infant's repertoire of responses does not immediately provide the means of control. The infant must learn to persist and to try alternatives. Therefore, once there is evidence that the contingent response is used generally to control various toys and events, a new contingency is introduced. Fig 4 shows the behavior of an infant with Down syndrome responding to a leg contingency after having initially learned an arm contingency. Fig 4 shows that the second contingency introduced to control a novel toy was learned within the session. The arm response, which was dominant in the first 3 minutes, was eventually suppressed.

Concept 5: Concept 3 revisited—Generalizing the new response to various consequences

Consistent with our desire to ensure that the new response is one that the infant uses as a general means of controlling events, a novel toy was introduced when

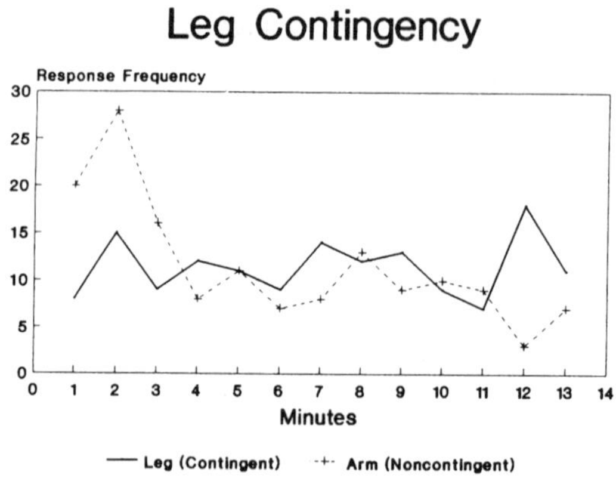

Fig 4. Initial response of an infant with Down syndrome subsequent to training with an arm contingency.

habituation occurred, and evidence for recovery of the appropriate response was sought. Because the infant had experienced two different means of controlling outcomes in the contingency intervention environment, a change in toys presented a real problem-solving event. In this setting, the infant may persist with the new contingent response because that has been successful most recently (an essentially conservative strategy known as win-stay), or the infant may choose to explore the formerly contingent response, resorting to a familiar method in the face of change (resorting to an old habit).

Fig 5 shows the behavior of one 7-month-old infant with Down syndrome to this contingency problem. Fig 5 is particularly striking because it shows that the infant made a left-right discrimination, which in our experience is a more difficult problem than arm-leg discrimination. We typically work with the right arm as the initial contingency (unless there is good reason not to) because the majority of infants tend to have a right hand bias for arm responses. In this particular child's contingency intervention experience, a left arm contingency was introduced after both arm and leg contingencies had been mastered. In this, the third contingent response to be introduced, both the right arm (initial contingent response) and the left arm (most recent contingent response) were available, and the infant's task was to choose the appropriate response both initially and after the toy change. Fig 5 shows that the infant chose the appropriate response for both toys.

Concept 6: Exploring ("Responses are tools for making things happen")

To this point we have focused on teaching separately two different responses that control various events. The infant has learned to persist with a response as

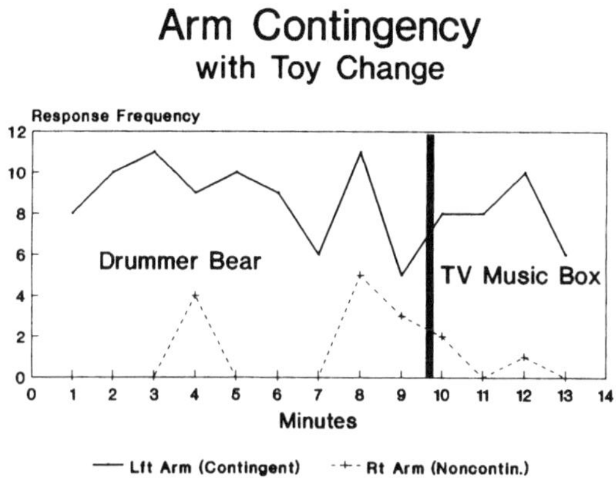

Fig 5. Recovery of left arm response by a 7-month-old infant in response to a toy change.

long as it continues to result in interesting outcomes. Now, the infant must experience shifting between responses at its disposal when appropriate. The means used to control environmental ends must be used flexibly as situations demand; the infant must shift to other responses when one does not work and must explore among the responses in its repertoire to play and engage environments outside the contingency intervention environment. We already have taught the infant the win-stay strategy; we now also teach the infant a lose-shift strategy. The consequence of not shifting is anger and frustration when the infant encounters contexts in which the response that made the world work does not work any longer.[32] To promote this strategy, we switch the switch. The session begins with a familiar response and familiar contingent outcome that the infant has already learned and enjoys. Midsession, without signal, the entire contingency switches; a different response and a different outcome go into effect, and the original contingency retires. The different contingency consists of a familiar response that has been used to control toys (the toy may or may not be novel). The infant is now asked to discover that the rules of the contingency game have changed, however, and to shift appropriately from one means of control to another.

Fig 6 shows an infant successfully accomplishing this task. In the 6 minutes of the session, tapping on a plate switch controlled a musical jack-in-the-box and a roller (also sometimes called a barrel switch) was the noncontingent response being monitored. After 6 minutes, the contingency was shifted to the roller, which controlled a musical cymbal-playing bear. The tap switch continued to be monitored. The result was a shift from one means to another, and the infant successfully remained in control of an interesting outcome. This type of response usually took several sessions to emerge in the infants we studied.

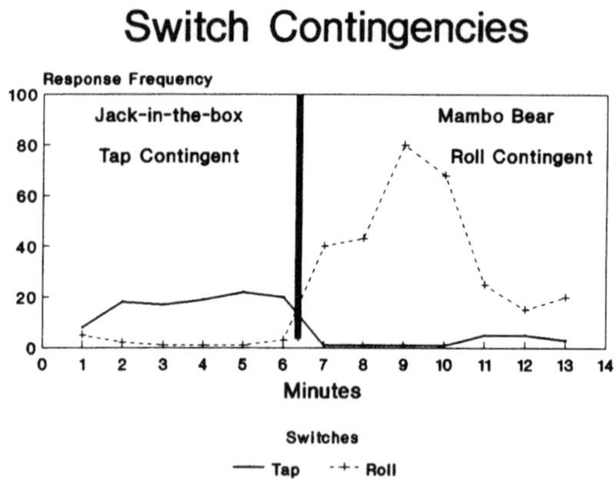

Fig 6. Change in switch use in response to a change in contingency.

WHERE THE CURRICULUM ENDS

Not all infants in the field study mastered all the levels of the program in the 3-month intervention period, and the time needed to master each level was highly variable across infants. Some of the concepts were mastered in what appeared to be a single session, whereas others took a significant portion of the 3-month program. A few infants with profound motor disabilities never progressed beyond the first concepts of contingency awareness. Some learned to shift responses flexibly, but others could not in the time allotted. What seems important, however, is not the exact proportion of the sample or any particular disability type that progressed through the program but that any infants were able to learn at all. Infants with various levels of motor and cognitive deficits learned control of simple outcomes by using methods that have been studied in the laboratory with normal infants and within short periods of time.

The inescapable conclusion of the project is that the majority of disabled infants younger than 15 months passed beyond the most basic level of contingency awareness and appeared to generalize their responses to other stimuli. They showed this ability despite the fact that their motor disabilities provided limited opportunity to do so in the everyday environment and despite cognitive delays. Even when these infants failed to master a concept, they made predictable errors, such as choosing a previously successful response. Few, if any, infants responded in a totally random fashion or failed to become excited and activated by contingency experiences.

The implication of these results is that some type of systematic contingency curriculum that uses technology should be a component of infant intervention. If motivation, attention, and fostering of engagement of the physical environment are considered important goals for the disabled infant, then switches, adapted toys, and other currently available technologies are the tools for achieving these goals and can be introduced at levels of cognitive functioning as early as 2 to 3 months. We have developed a curriculum of contingency activities that use switch-toy technology appropriate for this developmental level. If infants and toddlers can master the problems provided here, there is no reason that they cannot eventually use switch-toys for receptive speech activities and, ultimately, use a switch-adapted computer for educational and leisure activities. Indeed, a number of the infants in the project, now in preschool, have made this transition successfully. Some disabled infants may not need to rely on technology as they develop. Infants with Down syndrome and mild cerebral palsy may well outgrow switch-toy technology, whereas other infants will be dependent on assistive devices all their lives.

If one wishes to avoid learned helplessness in these children, contingency intervention must begin as early as possible. Even for the most profoundly impaired infants, provision of electronic playpens or activity centers—contingency play environments in which infants may learn to play and choose—might lead ultimately to the development of better generalization of skills. Even in the short term, as we have shown, this can lead to improved attention and enjoyment on the part of the child and a belief on the part of parents that learning is possible for their disabled infant. For these reasons, technology in infant intervention is warranted.

REFERENCES

1. Behrman MM, Jones TK, Wilds ML, Technology intervention for very young children with disabilities. *Infants Young Child.* 1989;1(4):66–77.
2. Lancioni GE. Infant operant conditioning and its implications for early intervention. *Psychol Bull.* 1980;88:546–554.
3. DeVellis RF, McCauley C. Perception of contingency and mental retardation. *Autism Dev Disord.* 1979;9:261–270.
4. Brinker R, Lewis M. Contingency intervention in infancy. In: Anderson J, ed. *Curricula for High Risk and Handicapped Infants.* Chapel Hill, NC: Technical Assistance and Development System, University of North Carolina; 1982:37–41.
5. Brinker R, Lewis M. Discovering the competent handicapped infant: a process approach to assessment and intervention. *Top Early Child Spec Educ.* 1982;2:1–16.
6. Brinker R, Lewis M. Making the world work with microcomputers: a learning prosthesis for handicapped infants. *Except Child.* 1982;49:163–169.
7. Maier SF, Seligman MEP. Learned helplessness: theory and evidence. *J Exp Psychol Gen.* 1976;105:3–46.
8. Seligman MEP. *On Helplessness, Depression and Death.* San Francisco, Calif: Freeman; 1975.
9. Rothbaum F. Children's clinical syndromes and generalized expectations of control. In: Reese HW, Lipsitt LP, eds. *Advances in Child Development and Behavior.* New York, NY: Academic Press; 1980;15:207–246.

10. Sigel IE. Application of research to psycho-educational treatment of infants at risk. In: Kearsely RB, Sigel IE, eds. *Infants at Risk: Assessment of Cognitive Functioning.* Hillsdale, NJ: Erlbaum; 1979;205–217.
11. Bandura A. Self-efficacy: toward a unifying theory of behavioral change. *Psychol Rev.* 1977;84:191–215.
12. White RW. Motivation reconsidered: the concept of competence. *Psychol Rev.* 1959;66:297–323.
13. Piaget J. *The Origins of Intelligence in Children.* New York, NY: International Universities Press; 1952.
14. Uzgiris IC, Hunt JV. *Assessment in Infancy: Ordinal Scales of Psychological Development.* Chicago, Ill: University of Chicago Press; 1976.
15. Dunst CJ. *A Clinical and Educational Manual for Use with the Uzgiris and Hunt Scales of Infant Psychological Development.* Austin, Tex: Pro-Ed; 1980.
16. Lewis M, Sullivan M, Brooks-Gunn J. Emotional behavioral during the learning contingency in early infancy. *Br J Dev Psychol.* 1985;3:307–316.
17. Watson J. Smiling, cooing and "the game." *Merrill-Palmer Q* 1972;17:139–152.
18. Millar WS. Smiling, vocal and attentive behavior in 7 and 10-month-old infants. *Merrill-Palmer Q.* 1988;34:301–325.
19. Sullivan MW, Lewis M. Facial expressions during learning in one-year-olds. *Infant Behav Dev.* 1988;11:373–377.
20. Rovee-Collier CK, Fagen J. A conditioning analysis of infant memory: how do we know that they know what we know they know? In: Isaacson RL, Spears NE, eds. *The Experience of Knowing.* New York, NY: Plenum; 1982;1–55.
21. Sullivan MW, Rovee-Collier CK, Tynes DM. A conditioning analysis of long-term memory in 3-month-old infants. *Child Dev.* 1979;50:152–162.
22. Alessandri SM, Sullivan MW, Lewis M. Violation of expectancy and frustration in early infancy. *Dev Psychol.* 1990;26:738–744.
23. Millar WS. *The Use of Noncontingent Stimulation in Infant Learning Research.* In press.
24. Gunnar MR. Control, warning signals, and distress in infancy. *Child Dev.* 1980;16:281–289.
25. Lewis M, Goldberg S. Perceptual-cognitive development in infancy: a generalized expectancy model as a function of the mother-infant interaction. *Merrill-Palmer Q.* 1969;15:81–100.
26. Lewis M, Coates DL. Mother-infant interactions and cognitive development in twelve-week-old infants. *Infant Behav Dev.* 1980;3:95–105.
27. Lewis M, Freedle R. Mother-infant dyad: the cradle of meaning. In: Pliner P, Krames L, Alloway T, eds. *Communication and Affect: Language and Thought.* New York, NY: Academic Press; 1973:127–155.
28. Dunham PJ, Hurshman F, Alexander T. Social contingency effects on subsequent perceptual cognitive tasks in young infants. *Child Dev.* 1989;60:1486–1496.
29. Dunham P, Dunham F. Effects of mother-infant social interactions on infant's subsequent contingency performance. *Child Dev.* 1990;61:785–793.
30. Lewis M, Rosenblum L. *The Effect of the Infant on its Caregiver: The Origins of Behavior.* New York, NY: Wiley. 1974;1.
31. Sullivan M, Lewis M. Emotion and cognition in infancy: facial expressions during contingency learning. *Int Behav Dev.* 1989;12:221–237.
32. Lewis M, Alessandri S, Sullivan MW. Violation of expectancy, loss of control, and anger in young infants. *Dev Psychol.* 1990;26:745–751.

33. Gekoski MJ, Rovee-Collier CK, Carulli-Rabinowitz V. A longitudinal analysis of inhibition of infant distress: the origins of social expectations. *Infant Behav Dev.* 1983;6:339–351.

34. Ohr P, Fagen JW. Learning and memory in infants with Down syndrome. *Am J Ment Defic.* 1991;96:151–162.

35. Fagen JW, Rovee-Collier CK. Effects of quantitative shifts in a visual reinforcer on the instrumental response of infants. *J Exp Child Psychol.* 1976;21:346–360.

36. Rovee-Collier CK. Learning and memory in infancy. In: Osofsky JD, ed. *Handbook of Infant Development* (2nd ed). New York, NY: Wiley; 1987.

37. Rovee-Collier CK, Sullivan MW. Organization of infant memory. *J Exp Psychol Hum Learn Mem.* 1982;6:798–807.

38. Rovee-Collier CK, Patterson J, Hayne H. Specificity in the reactivation of infant memory. *Dev Psychol.* 1985;18:559–574.

39. Sullivan MW. Reactivation: priming forgotten memories in human infants. *Child Dev.* 1982;53:516–523.

40. Rovee-Collier CK, Sullivan MW, Lucas D, Fagen J. Reactivation of infant memory. *Science.* 1980;208:1159–1161.

41. Butler J, Rovee-Collier CK. Contextual gating of memory retrieval. *Dev Psychol.* 1989;22:533–552.

42. Fagen JF, Morrongiello B, Rovee-Collier CK, Gekoski MJ. Expectancies and memory retrieval in 3-month-old infants. *Child Dev.* 1984;48:786–796.

43. Rovee-Collier CK, Greisler PC, Early L. Contextual determinants of retrieval in three-month-old infants. *Learn Motiv.* 1985;16:139–157.

44. Rovee-Collier CK, DuFault D. Multiple contexts and memory retrieval at 3 months. *Dev Psychobiol.* In press.

45. Sameroff AJ, Cavanagh PJ. Learning in infancy: a developmental perspective. In: Osofsky J, ed. *Handbook of Infant Development.* New York, NY: Wiley; 1979:344–392.

46. Rovee-Collier CK, Morrongiello B, Aron M, Kuperschmidt J. Topographical response differentiation and reversal in 3-month-old infants. *Infant Behav Dev.* 1978;1:323–333.

47. Fagen JW, Rovee-Collier CK, Kaplan MG. Psychophysical scaling of stimulus similarity in 3-month-old infants and adults. *J Exp Child Psychol.* 1976;22:272–281.

48. Timmons R. *Interaction of Codependent Memories in 6-Month-Old Infants.* New Brunswick, NJ: Rutgers University; 1991. Thesis.

49. Sullivan MW, Lewis M, Alessandri S. Cross-age stability in emotional expressions during learning and extinction. *Dev Psychol.* 1992;28:58–63.

50. Dunst CJ, Cushing PJ, Vance SD. Response contingent learning in profoundly handicapped infants: a social systems perspective. *Anal Intervent Dev Disabil.* 1985;5:33–47.

51. Sullivan MW, Lewis M. Contingency intervention: a program portrait. *J Early Intervent.* 1990;14:367–375.

52. Utley B, Duncan D, Strain P, Scalon K. Effects of contingent and noncontingent vision stimulation in multiply handicapped children. *TASH J.* 1983;8:29–42.

53. Brinker RP. The microcomputer as perceptual tool: search for systematic learning strategies with handicapped infants. In: Bennett RE, Maher CA, eds. *Microcomputers and Exceptional Children: Special Services in the Schools.* New York, NY: Haworth; 1984.

Incorporating computer technology into activity-based thematic units for young children with disabilities

Moira A. Fallon, PhD
Assistant Professor

Jennifer A. Sanders Wann, MA, CCC-SLP
Lecturer
Department of Special Education
Murray State University
Murray, Kentucky

PROFESSIONALS from a variety of disciplines agree that the best environments for all young children are natural environments that encourage active learning, utilize concrete manipulatives, are creative, and allow for problem solving.[1–6] The introduction of computer technology into early childhood classrooms was meant to enhance these ideal properties of early childhood programs. Some educational research has theorized that the use of technology can have a major impact upon children's understanding of the relationship between cause and effect in the daily environment.[7]

Parette[8] suggests that the use of technology can enable young children with special needs to more successfully explore the world around them, to communicate their needs to others, and to make choices about their world. Necessary developmental skills affected by the disability are best taught in a natural environment. Once taught, practice of developmental skills within a social environment is critical. Without this foundation, generalization to other environments is impossible. Therefore, the ideal environment for young children with disabilities is one in which they can both consistently practice and generalize their learning, such as in an inclusive social environment.

Inclusion is defined as the placement of children with disabilities in regular education programs to the maximum extent possible so that they can reach their fullest potential.[9] Although regular education teachers, along with special education professionals, have begun to serve young children with disabilities in these natural settings, many suggest that the use of computer technology is necessary for full inclusion. Teachers can utilize technology to remediate or circumvent the disability and allow these children equal access to classroom activities.

Unfortunately, some professionals state that computer use has been incidental in preschool classrooms.[2,10] They suggest that computer use is often restricted to drill and practice, especially for lower functioning children. It is essential that professionals think carefully about the preschool classroom environment and its relationship to computer technology in an inclusive preschool classroom. The remainder of this article will discuss practical techniques for incorporating computer technology into activity-based thematic units for use in an inclusive preschool classroom.

Inf Young Children 1994; 6(4): 64–69

TECHNIQUES FOR INCORPORATING COMPUTER TECHNOLOGY INTO ACTIVITY-BASED THEMATIC UNITS

The building of any activity-based thematic unit incorporating computer technology for use in an inclusive preschool classroom must include four steps: building an activity-based thematic unit, choosing appropriate software, individualizing activities extending computer learning, and implementing instruction. Each step is critical, with none being more or less important than the other; balance among these steps is essential. Each step and its relationship to the other three steps will be discussed in turn. Furthermore, an activity-based thematic unit on body parts for use in an inclusive preschool classroom will be provided as an example.

Step 1: Building an activity-based thematic unit

Bricker and Cripe[11] state that activity-based thematic units can be an effective curricular strategy for organizing and supporting group learning. They outline an activity-based thematic unit with four components: an initial description or sequence to the theme, variations within the theme, materials used, and instructional objectives. When developing an activity-based thematic unit, begin with a team approach to the selection of a theme. Our team consisted of a special educator, a regular educator, a speech-language pathologist, and a physical therapist. The concept of "All About Me!" was chosen as our example of a theme. Appendix A contains our sample activity-based thematic unit.

Our goal was to facilitate the learning of the various body parts, beginning with the face. We decided that our thematic description/sequence should include identifying and naming the facial features, such as eyes, ears, or nose, first; followed by the primary body parts, such as arms, legs, hands, and stomach; and then the secondary body parts, such as fingers, wrist, or knee. Once the sequence has been generally outlined, the next step is to conceptualize ways in which we might vary the theme. We decided that these variations would include identifying and naming body parts on self and peers and on dolls or other inanimate objects, and constructing a face and body "from scratch."

Our materials included dolls and stuffed animals, puzzles, Mr. Potato Head, books, flannelboard games, and art materials for drawing and constructing body parts. We then wrote general instructional objectives by domains. The purpose of these objectives was to focus our teaching instruction on what the children in our inclusive classroom needed to learn. Although instructional objectives will differ for the individual needs of each classroom, Appendix A contains a sample of instructional objectives we used in our setting. The next step is to match appropriate software to the activity-based thematic unit general outline.

Step 2: Choosing appropriate software

The software for an activity-based thematic unit must be carefully chosen. Selection of the software program is an important link between the computer learning and the generalization of learning to other classroom activities. Simply utilizing a software program whose subject matter is the same as the thematic unit is insufficient to significantly improve learning. Some professionals state that the most appropriate software encourages creativity and socialization among children; allows children to work at a functional level; and generalizes to new settings, objects, and people.[1,4]

In determining an appropriate software program for our unit, we began by reviewing a variety of software programs whose purpose was to teach body parts. We believed we could best implement our activity-based thematic unit using the *Facemaker Golden Edition.*[12] We had specifically looked for a program that sequentially taught the levels of body parts outlined in our unit so that the children could progress in their learning. We also wanted a program that allowed the children to practice their skills without adult supervision or aid. We facilitated that independence by color coding the important keys on the keyboard. *Facemaker* had the additional advantage of teaching an action for each body part, such as making the mouth smile by simply pressing the appropriate key. Our next step was to develop classroom activities that would extend what *Facemaker* taught to concrete manipulatives in the natural environment.

Step 3: Activities to generalize computer learning

The selection, design, and implementation of activities to generalize computer learning is also a vital component of the process. Children need the chance to practice, apply, and extend their computer learning. Balancing these activities with the computer instruction can significantly improve children's learning and application of that learning to new settings and objects. We approached the selection and design of these activities carefully.

We believed it was important for classroom activities to be relevant to the classroom setting and the individual needs of our students. In addition, these activities must follow the activity-based theme. As with the selection of software, the activities must lend themselves to generalization to new settings beyond the computer lesson. They must be concrete, developmentally appropriate, natural, and allow for hands-on manipulation for children. Finally, the activities must allow for children to work at a variety of functional levels. We designed several activities for our sample activity-based thematic unit. Examples of two activities can be found in Appendix B.

Step 4: Implementation of the activity-based thematic unit

The instructional methods used in implementing the activity-based thematic unit will depend in a large part on the individual classroom needs. In general, the instructional implementation of an activity-based thematic unit should approximate the learning process that occurs naturally in children. The teacher's role in facilitating this process is to first introduce the program to the children. After initial demonstration by the teacher, the children have the opportunity for hands-on individual manipulation. During this time, the teacher provides opportunities for participation at the children's levels of ability.

In our sample thematic unit, the group instruction took place during the morning circle time. The classroom activities designed to extend computer learning followed during learning center time. Members of the team facilitated this extension at the various centers, modeling and following the childrens' lead in play. We made specific adaptations in both group and individual instruction for children who were physically, hearing, and visually impaired. To implement a truly inclusive classroom, teachers may have to adapt the computer for some children's needs. It is beyond the scope of this article to provide extensive information regarding computer adaptation options for specific disabilities. Currently, there are a variety of projects designed to aid professionals in this area, including the Los Angeles Unified School District/University of California, Los Angeles (LAUSD/UCLA) Microcomputer Project,[13] the Preschool Integration Through Technology Systems (PITTS) Project,[14] and Project Activating Children Through Technology (ACTT).[15] Other suggestions for accessing technology training include finding out about local computer user groups; enrolling in college courses using computers; and subscribing to newsletters, magazines, and journals such as *Closing the Gap* (P.O. Box 68, Henderson, MN, 56044).[16]

• • •

Inclusion of young children with disabilities can be effective if various factors are addressed. The success of teaching children inclusively rather than in isolation lies in the integration of instructional objectives, the careful selection of software with appropriate instructional design features, and generalization of computer instruction across other classroom activities. In our sample activity-based thematic unit, we found that not only was computer instruction a collaborative effort among all the children participating, but the selection and implementation of activities to generalize computer learning made inclusion truly successful.

REFERENCES

1. Clements D, Natasi B, Swaminathan S. Young children and computers: crossroads and directions from research. *Young Child.* 1993;48(2):56–64.
2. Davidson J. Computers for preschoolers? *Pre-K Today.* 1988;2(5):28–29.
3. Lewis RB. *Special Education Technology: Classroom Applications.* Pacific Grove, Calif: Brooks/Cole Publishing; 1993.
4. Beatty JJ, Tucker WH. *The Computer as a Paintbrush: Creative Uses for the Personal Computer in the Preschool Classroom.* Columbus, Ohio: Merrill Publishing; 1987.
5. Fazio B, Polsgrove L. An evaluation of training special educators to integrate microcomputer technology into math curricula. *J Spec Educ Technol.* 1989;10(2):5–13.
6. Bredekamp S, ed. *Developmentally Appropriate Practice in Early Childhood Programs Serving Children from Birth Through Age 8: Expanded Edition.* Washington, DC: National Association for the Education of Young Children; 1992.
7. Brinker R, Lewis M. Making the world work with microcomputers: a learning prosthesis for handicapped infants. *Except Child.* 1982;49(2):163–170.
8. Parette H, ed. *Assistive Technology Guide for Young Children With Disabilities: A Planning for State Technology Service Delivery.* Little Rock, Ark: Arkansas Governor's Developmental Disabilities Planning Council; 1990.
9. Viadero D. All together now: schools bring disabled children into regular classrooms. *Teacher Mag.* 1993;January:10–12.
10. McCarthy R. Making the future work: the road to curriculum integration. *Electronic Learning.* 1988;8(1):42–46.
11. Bricker D, Cripe J. *An Activity-Based Approach to Early Intervention.* Baltimore, Md: Paul Brookes; 1992.
12. *Facemaker Golden Edition.* Cambridge, Mass: Spinnaker Software Corporation; 1986.
13. *Computer Use for Special Needs Children: An Instructional Guide for Families and Professionals.* Los Angeles, Calif: Los Angeles Unified School District/UCLA Intervention Program; 1993.
14. *Preschool Integration Through Technology Systems (PITTS).* Buffalo,NY: United Cerebral Palsy Association of Western New York; 1993.
15. *Activating Children Through Technology (ACTT).* Macomb, Ill: Macomb Projects, College of Education, Western Illinois University; 1993.
16. Armstrong JS, Jones K. *Getting off to a great start: Using assistive technology with young children.* Presented at the Closing the Gap Conference; Minneapolis, Minn; October 1993.

Appendix A: Sample Activity-Based Thematic Unit

Name of Unit: All About Me!

Objectives by Domains:

Gross Motor: kinesthetic awareness
Fine Motor: reach, grasp, and manipulation of objects
Cognition: awareness of body parts
Communication: receptive and expressive knowledge of body parts
Social: turn-taking, joint awareness, verbal and gestural interaction

Description:

Identify body parts, beginning with facial features such as eye, nose, mouth, hair, and ears. Have the children watch while the teacher points to the body parts. Have the children point to the same body parts on each other. Name the body parts while the children imitate. Ask "What's this?" while pointing to body parts. Tickle or use textures to touch body parts. Proceed to a demonstration of hand, arm, leg, foot, head, chest, back, and tummy. Repeat modeling, pointing to body parts on each other and naming body parts. Demonstrate secondary body parts such as finger, toe, wrist, knee, and elbow. Repeat modeling, pointing, and naming.

Variations:

1. Have the children point to and name body parts on themselves using a mirror.
2. Use dolls and stuffed animals for expressive and receptive knowledge of body parts.
3. Sing "Head, Shoulders, Knees and Toes" or play the "Hokey Pokey" with children.
4. Trace around children while they are lying on a piece of paper. Allow the children to color and decorate themselves.
5. Read books such as *Bath Time for John* or *I Like Me!*

Materials:

Mr. Potato Head, books, flannelboard, art materials (crayons, paper, scissors, paint, and brushes), dolls and stuffed animals, puzzles, books

Appendix B: Sample Activities to Generalize Computer Learning

Mr. Potato Head

Materials: Mr. Potato Head(s)
Play-Doh
Play-Doh tools

Procedure: Introduce the Mr. Potato Head with all of the pieces in the heads. First instruct the children to remove all the eyes. Take out each piece one by one and then let the children put them back in as they wish.

Variations: After the children have learned how to use the Mr. Potato Heads, introduce some Play-Doh and some tools to make hair for the heads. Children can also make hats and the various facial features with the Play-Doh. Have plastic knives available to cut the Play-Doh.

Adaptations: For children with motor impairments, use any type of adhesive to attach the head onto the table so the child will not have to hold the toy while putting pieces in or taking pieces out.

Drawing Faces

Materials: Chalk board
Chalk
Erasers
Magna Doodle

Procedure: Encourage the children to draw faces. Ask each child to draw another child's face ("Draw Amy"). Praise any markings ("Oh, look, it's Amy."). The adult can take turns drawing children. "Who is this?" the teacher can ask. Praise any answer. Ask a child to draw someone but NOT to tell who. "Guess" who they drew (*Hint:* They will usually be looking right at the person they drew.)

Variations: Use chalk boards but no chalk, just water. The children will have to guess who was drawn before the water dries!

Adaptations: For children with motor impairments, attach a magnet onto a dowel or head stick for use with the Magna Doodle.

The use of videotaping in the evaluation of preschool-aged children and their parents

Ira Glovinsky, PhD
Co-Director, Early Childhood Program
Center for Human Development
William Beaumont Hospital
Royal Oak, Michigan

WITHIN THE LAST TWO decades there has been an increasing effort to develop ways to evaluate parent–child interactions. Beginning with a focus on cognitive and motor development, assessment has now extended to the socioemotional arena and to wider family interactions.

Moving away from pure research for the purpose of studying infant development, investigators have begun to focus on assessing parent–child interactions for the purpose of identifying potential interactive problems and developing appropriate and effective intervention programs. Public Law 99-457, which amended Public Law 94-142, emphasizes the development of an Individualized Family Service Plan (IFSP) to help families with disabled or handicapped infants and toddlers. Thus, assessment of parent–child interactions is a core component of developing services for families identified as having special needs.

Videotaping parent–child interactions has facilitated understanding of dyadic interactions. Microanalytic techniques of analyzing videotaped interactions have opened a window to understanding how relationships develop.[1–3] Videotaping has taken different forms depending on the age of the child. With younger infants, feeding interactions, face-to-face interactions, and perturbations of face-to-face interactions have been used. As children get older and more motoric, floor play, teaching interactions, and attachment interactions have been studied.[4]

Videotapes of infants and toddlers and their parents are helping to identify potentially problematic interaction patterns. For example, videotapes have been useful in identifying infants who do not initiate facial expressions or who do not show facial expressiveness, thus making it difficult for parents to read their emotions.[5-7] Videotapes have also helped to identify serious psychopathology such as the early stages in the development of autism.[8]

Within recent years the use of videotapes in clinical settings has increased. The proliferation of research in videotaping as a therapeutic tool has resulted in the publication of several books.[9-11] Videotaping has been used in clinical settings where infants and parents are evaluated for intervention. In this article the use of videotapes in evaluating infants, toddlers, and preschool-aged children in a clinical setting will be described.

The author thanks Dr Susan McDonough, Dr Richard Galpin, Dr Karen Mikus, Dr Jack Heckerl, Cindy Glovinsky, and Linda Frauenheim for their help in preparing this article.

Inf Young Children 1993; 6(2): 60–66

Examples of the use of videotapes in clinical settings have begun to appear in the literature. Greenspan and Lieberman[12] developed the Greenspan-Lieberman Observational Scale (GLOS), in which mothers and infants interact in an unstructured 10-minute play situation that is videotaped. The videotape is then scored for a number of variables at 15-second intervals to develop a profile of parent–infant interactions. Clark and Seifer[13] have also developed a technique and a scale to assess interaction styles in parents and their infants.

Recently, Stern-Bruschweiler and Stern[14] described the use of videotaping in a psycho-educational model that has been named "interactional coaching." In this model, a mother is asked to interact in an unstructured play situation with her child; the interaction is videotaped. Immediately after the play session, which generally lasts about 10 minutes, the mother and the therapist review the tape. The videotaped interaction then becomes the source and the content of the therapeutic interaction. The treatment focuses on the mother's behavior and attempts to alter it when the interaction between the mother and the infant is maladaptive. As the mother's behavior changes there is a corresponding change in the infant's behavior. In addition, by selecting positive parent behaviors for discussion, the therapist attempts to increase the mother's self-esteem. This increase in self-esteem in turn results in a change in the mother's internal representation of herself vis-à-vis the infant. Changes in maternal behavior and the mother's internal representation of her child not only contribute to changes in the infant's behavior but also, over time, begin to change the representation that the infant is developing of himself or herself and his or her mother. In interactional coaching, positive reinforcement is stressed. In addition, giving the parent information and advice is important; interpretation is not used.

McDonough[15] developed an "interactional guidance model" to work with multiproblem, multirisk families. Videotaping is an important component of this model in which family members interact in an unstructured family–infant play session. Approximately 6 minutes of the play session are taped and this tape becomes the "movie" that the family and the therapist watch following family–infant play. This video segment is discussed by family members with the therapist.

The author's videotaping model is a form of interactional coaching that involves both parents and their child. It is being used in assessing parent–child interactions and then in treating infants, toddlers, and their parents.

EVALUATION OF CHILDREN AND PARENTS

The evaluation begins by having the father and the mother fill out a Behavioral Style Questionnaire[16] separately. The questionnaires are then scored prior to the initial intake in which parents discuss their concerns and present developmental and family information.

Approximately 1 week after the intake the referred child is seen for psychological testing. Depending on the child's age, the Bayley Scales of Infant Development,[17] the McCarthy Scales of Children's Abilities,[18] or the Wechsler Preschool and Primary Scale of Intelligence-Revised[19] is used.

Following the testing, a videotaping session is scheduled for approximately a week later. Each parent is videotaped with the child first using the Marschak Interaction Method,[20] and then using a 10-minute unstructured free play session, including cleaning up.

The Marschak is a structured play situation in which the parent and the child interact by performing a task that is presented on a color-coded index card. The colors reflect one of four categories: attachment, alert to environment, purposive behavior, and stress reduction. In videotaping sessions the author uses five or six tasks, each of which is taped for 3 minutes.

Following the videotaping, the parents are invited back to view the tape with the clinician who did the taping. Each play task is viewed by both parents, after which it is discussed. The videotape may be stopped at any point if the parent or clinician chooses to focus on a particular segment.

While viewing each parent–child interaction, it is important to point out positive aspects of the interaction to the parents. It is also essential to stress parental strengths and to promote feelings of success by providing positive reinforcement. Positive reinforcement is a central characteristic of "interactional coaching" procedures.[15]

Having both parents present to view the videotape is important, too. In addition to giving each parent the opportunity to view himself or herself with the child and to discuss the interaction, it gives both parents the opportunity to see how the child interacts with the other parent without the second parent present. In natural home situations when one parent observes the other parent with the child, it is automatically a triadic situation because both parents are present even if only one is interacting with the child. It is difficult to determine how the child perceives or interprets having both parents present at the same time. It is also difficult to determine how both parents being present influences the child's behavior. Thus, videotaping offers each parent the opportunity to see the child functioning in a dyadic interaction. Differences between dyadic interactions, in the videotaping, and triadic interactions, at home, can then be discussed.

Having both parents present also enables observation of parents' interactive and relating abilities. How does the couple work as a unit? What are their strengths and weaknesses individually and as a couple? What aspects or themes does each parent focus on? Are there perceptual "biases" or "readiness" evident?[21]

One can begin to determine the needs of the parents and what therapeutic approach might be undertaken if treatment is necessary. Finally, having both parents present and actively participating in the evaluation gives each spouse the signal that he or she is valued and is essential to the assessment and treatment process.

CASE PRESENTATION

Jim, age 20 months, was the youngest of four children, two boys and two girls. He was referred because of his parents' concerns about slow development in language functioning and gross motor functioning. He was not doing the things that the other toddlers in this mother–toddler program were doing.

Jim was a full-term baby, born after an uneventful pregnancy. No neonatal problems were reported. With the exception of a series of ear infections, he had been a healthy child.

The possibility of delays was first considered at the time Jim began to crawl. Unlike other infants or toddlers he was reluctant to roam about and seemed to always want to be held. When he did crawl he continually bumped into things and had numerous accidents. In addition, at age 20 months he was not yet using single words or making gestures to make his needs known.

Jim's parents described themselves as healthy, and there was no history of learning or emotional problems in the family.

DEVELOPMENTAL ASSESSMENT

The Functional Assessment Scale,[22] described by Greenspan, was used to evaluate Jim's level of functioning. He appeared to be weak in listening to sounds for 3+ seconds and to ignore auditory input even though a previous hearing evaluation indicated normal hearing.

Jim evidenced only a fleeting interest in his parents even when they were happy or assertive with him. He responded to social overtures with weak, intermittent smiles. For the most part, however, his behavioral responses were noncontingent. When either parent changed facial expression or vocalized there was a clear tendency toward gaze aversion. In addition, he did not smile at his mirror image.

There were no clear intentional behaviors or contingent responses to either parent. At 20 months, he was still neither initiating gestural signals nor responding to others' attempts to initiate social interaction. His emotional response was variable as he seemed to shift quickly from a low-keyed sober emotional pattern to intense laughter, and quickly back again.

On selected motor tasks Jim obtained scores within the 13- to-18-month age range; he was functioning within the same range in sensory functioning. Language development was significantly delayed; he received a "fleetingly present" rating for responding to his name, a 9-month level behavior (intentional two-way communication). Jim seemed content to play on his own for long periods of time and received credit for this cognitive item at the behavioral organization level of 13 months. On the Bayley Scales of Infant Development Jim evidenced significant delays; his highest passed item was approximately 5 months below his chronologic age level. He did not obtain credit for any language items.

VIDEOTAPING JIM AND HIS PARENTS

Jim was videotaped in a 30-minute session with his mother and then a 30-minute session with his father. For the first 15 minutes of each session five tasks from the Marschak Interaction Method were videotaped. Then each parent was told to play with Jim as if at home. Jim's parents were permitted to use any of the toys in the playroom. After the videotaping, the author reviewed the tape with Jim's parents. In order to illustrate how the videotape was used in this session, two tasks are discussed. In the first task, "Talking to Child," Jim's parents held him on their laps and talked to him.

Jim's mother held Jim in her lap facing her. She spoke in a rapid, staccato manner. As she spoke, Jim looked away. As he did, his mother moved her face closer to Jim in an attempt to capture his gaze. In response Jim became more actively avoidant, pushing backward and looking to one side. This "mother-chases-son gaze aversion" interaction was videotaped for 3 minutes.

When the videotape was reviewed in the follow-up visit Jim's mother immediately commented on Jim's difficulty in making eye-to-eye contact and her own frustration at not being able to engage him. In response, the author first reinforced Jim's mother for her attempts to keep trying, despite her obvious frustration. Then, picking up on her observation, the author began to talk with her about the attention-gaze aversion cycles that characterize younger infants' behaviors.[23] The discussion then focused on what would happen if Jim were allowed to avert eye gaze. Would he later attempt to re-engage spontaneously? Also discussed was the option of letting Jim take the lead and join in her play rather than attempting to lead her. Jim's mother spontaneously began to talk about her wish to talk to Jim. She recognized that she was overanxious and perhaps flooding Jim with words. The author then talked briefly about how painful it must be for her to experience Jim as turning away and how she might feel that it was her fault. The author pointed out how varied children are in their ability to process stimulation in different sensory modalities and that this variation was no one's fault.

When watching Jim's father in the same "talking task" some fleeting imitating behavior on Jim's part was observed as his father's vocal tone and pitch varied. Jim's facial expression briefly brightened to his father's "sing-song" vocal tone. Discussion thus focused on the value of "baby-talk" in interacting with a child who is functioning at a younger emotional level. Also discussed was the possibility of playing around with different kinds of auditory stimulation and different vocal tones to see to which Jim was more responsive.

In the second task, "Familiar Game," Jim's parents each initiated a game with him that they played at home. In a ball-rolling game Jim became quite animated as his mother rolled the ball to him. Fleeting contingent responses were observed as his mother called Jim to roll the ball back. Jim was suddenly more attentive. However, as mother became excited by his response and increased her demands, Jim again became noncontingent and averted his gaze. In viewing this on the screen, discussion focused on the parents' developmental expectations. Jim's mother was able to see that perhaps her expectations were unrealistic.

In his father's play interaction both parents observed Jim's immediate avoidance of rough-and-tumble play as contrasted with his ability to accept and even smile when he was moved rhythmically in a game of pat-a-cake. Both parents commented on the differences in their natural interactive styles. They were able to talk about the differences that they observed in Jim's responses. Talk then focused on the strengths of each style and how each parent could support and coach the other now that they saw things that seemed to evoke more positive, contingent responses in their son.

DEVELOPING A TREATMENT PLAN

The major outcome of the observation of the videotape was the development of a preliminary treatment plan that was essentially generated through the parents' spontaneous comments. Rather than imposing a plan on them, the plan that began to emerge was a natural outcome of what they were observing, thus, immediately making sense to them. The primary components of this preliminary plan included the following:

- Observing and timing Jim's attention-gaze aversion cycle and allowing him time to "distance behaviorally" without intruding on him.
- Engaging Jim by using physical contact rather than attempting to do so with words. After physical contact was made, words could be used to add multisensory stimulation, using playful variation of tone, pitch, and facial expression to increase attention.
- Using rhythmic play and limiting rough-and-tumble activities.
- Pairing inanimate stimuli with social stimuli to increase Jim's attention to his social environment. For example, while playing ball with Jim his parents could start by holding the ball to the side of their faces, creating the opportunity for Jim to establish eye-to-eye contact momentarily.
- Using sample phrases or single words in talking to Jim rather than using complex language that he probably was not able to process and that perhaps was even exacerbating his noncontingent responses.

DISCUSSION

Videotaping can be a valuable adjunct to parent–child assessment and intervention. First, it offers the parents the opportunity to observe themselves and their spouse with their child and then to discuss similarities and differences in their interactional styles. They can observe how they interact as well as the content of their interactions.

Observing interactions can also help parents develop a sense of a child's developmental level and the types of activities that might be above or below a child's capabilities. For example, Jim's parents were able to observe how difficult it was for Jim to understand them when they were using too many words. This response contrasted with his more positive responses to physical contact and rhythmic play.

Becoming aware of a child's capabilities in different developmental areas helps parents develop more appropriate behavioral expectations. Seeing a child's differential responses to varying levels or intensities of stimulation or expectations seems to be understood more quickly than simply talking about them. In effect, "A picture is worth a thousand words."

Another parent, viewing her child on the screen, exclaimed that when she is with her son he feels "so big" and his tantrums frighten her but when she saw him on the screen he seemed like such a little boy who needed help. Thus, even during an evaluation session, videotapes may begin to alter a parent's internal representation of the child, resulting in different behaviors toward the child in their interactions. This change may in turn begin to alter the child's developing internal representation of the parent and change interactions and the parent–child relationship.[14]

In viewing a videotape there is a wide range of visual and auditory stimulation on which a parent can focus. By waiting and allowing the parent to talk spontaneously he or she will signal the clinician as to what is most important to him or her. A parent, consciously or unconsciously, signals a moment of readiness and receptiveness. A spontaneous comment from a parent is often an invitation to the clinician, and the clinician can follow by expanding on the comment, exploring it further, and adding educational information. When a parent signals readiness, the follow-up input seems to be welcomed rather than perceived as criticism or an intrusion.

• • •

The videotaping model described in this article is being used in the evaluation procedure for infants, toddlers, and preschool-aged children. To date, it has been used with approximately 15 children and their parents. The author has found that using videotapes to focus on parent–child interactions enables parents to focus on their child's behaviors as well as on dyadic interactions between a parent and a child. Moreover, viewing behaviors on the screen facilitates altering parental responses to their child as they begin to recognize their child's strengths and weaknesses in interacting dyadically. Even during an evaluation, representations can begin to be altered on both the part of the child and the part of the parent. The model seems to facilitate the initiation of treatment, and changes occur within a short period of time. This finding is consistent with the conclusions of other investigators using interactional coaching methods.[9,10]

Experience with this model has also demonstrated that the boundary between assessment and treatment is a very blurry one. Assessment may in fact be a form of short-term treatment. When a parent meets with a clinician a relationship is established. A clinician must be aware of this. As a clinician interacts with a parent, the parent has his or her own definition of the meaning of the interaction. A parent in need listens very carefully to what is being said in order to extract something of importance that will make an immediate change. No parent wants to leave an appointment empty handed. Thus while the clinician may define the interaction as an assessment process, the parent may define it as an opportunity for help. The fact that changes can already be seen during an evaluation process indicates that evaluation is a form of intervention, and often an intervention that makes a significant impact on a parent–child relationship. Clinicians should therefore not overlook the importance of assessment as a form of intervention.

REFERENCES

1. Tronick E, Als H, Adamson L, Wise SE, Brazelton TB. The infant's response to entrapment and between contradictory messages in face-to-face interaction. *J Child Psychiatry.* 1978;17:1–13.
2. Beebe B, Jeff J, Feldstein S, Mays K, Alson D. Interpersonal timing: the application of an adult dialogue mood to mother–infant vocal kinesthetic interactions. In: Field T, Fox N, eds. *Social Perception in Infants.* Norwood, NJ: Ablex; 1985.
3. Cohen JF, Tronick EZ. Mother–infant face-to-face interactions: influence is bidirectional and unrelated to periodic cycles in either partner's behavior. *Dev Psychol.* 1988;24:382–389.
4. Field T. Assessment of parent–child interactions. In: Schaefer CE, Gitlin K, Sandgrund A, eds. *Play Diagnosis and Assessment.* New York, NY: Wiley, 1991.
5. Field T, Woodson R, Cohen D, Greenberg R, Garcia R, Collins D. Discrimination and imitation of facial expression by term and preterm neonates. *Inf Behav Dev.* 1983;6:485–490.
6. Field T. The 3Rs of infant–adult interaction. *J Pediatr Psychol.* 1978;3:131–136.
7. Goldberg S. Premature birth consequences for parent–infant relationship. *Am Scientist.* 1979;67:214–220.
8. Massie NH. Pathological interactions in infancy. In: Field TM, Goldberg S, Stein D, Sostek AM, eds. *High Risk Infants and Children: Adult and Peer Interactions.* New York, NY: Academic Press; 1980.
9. Berger MM, ed. *Videotaping Techniques in Psychiatric Training and Treatment.* 2nd ed. New York, NY: Brunner/Mazel; 1978.
10. Dowrick PW, Biggs SJ, eds. *Using Video: Psychological and Social Applications.* Chichester, United Kingdom: Wiley; 1983.
11. Dowrick PW. *Practical Guide in Using Video in Behavioral Sciences.* New York, NY: Wiley; 1991.
12. Greenspan S, Lieberman A. Infants, mothers and their interaction: a quantitative clinical approach to developmental assessment. In: Greenspan S, Pollock GH, eds. *The Course of Life: Psychoana-*

lytic Contributions toward Understanding Personality Development. Vol. 1; Infancy and Early Childhood. Adelphi, Md: NIMH; 1980.

13. Clark GN, Seifer R. Facilitating mother-infant communication: a treatment model for high-risk and developmentally delayed infants. *Inf Ment Health J.* 1983;4:67–82.
14. Stern-Bruschweiler N, Stern DN. A model for conceptualizing the role of mother's representational world in various mother–infant therapies. *Inf Ment Health J.* 1980;10:142–156.
15. McDonough SC. Interaction guidance: understanding and treating early infant–caregiver relationship disturbances. In: Zeanah CH, ed. *Handbook of Infant Mental Health.* New York, NY: Guilford Press; 1993.
16. McDevitt SC, Carey WB. *Behavioral Style Questionnaire.* Media, Pa: 1975.
17. Bayley N. *Bayley Scales of Infant Development.* Cleveland, Ohio: Psychological Corporation 1969.
18. McCarthy DA. *McCarthy Scales of Children's Abilities.* New York, NY: Psychological Corporation; 1972.
19. Wechsler D. *Wechsler Preschool and Primary Scale of Intelligence-Revised.* New York, NY: Psychological Corporation; 1989.
20. Jernberg A, Booth P, Koller T, Albert A. *Manual for the Administration and Clinical Interpretation of the Marschak Interaction Method: Preschool and School Age.* Chicago, Ill: The Theraplay Institute; 1987.
21. Malatesta CZ. The role of emotions in the development and organization of personality. In: Thompson R, ed. *Socioemotional Development.* Lincoln, Neb: Nebraska Symposium on Motivation; 1989.
22. Greenspan S. *Infancy and Early Childhood: The Practice of Clinical Assessment and Intervention with Emotional and Developmental Challenges.* Madison, Conn: 1992.
23. Brazelton TB, Koslowski B, Main M. The origins of reciprocity: early mother–infant interaction. In: Lewis M, Rosenblum L, eds. *The Effect of the Infant on Its Caregiver.* New York, NY: Wiley; 1974.

Written materials and the client with low literacy skills

Karen S. Edmondson, MN
Infant-Toddler Specialist
Developmental Evaluation Center
Asheville, North Carolina

Janyce J. Spell, PhD
Infant-Toddler Specialist
Development Evaluation Center
Cullowhee, North Carolina

WRITTEN MATERIALS represent a major mode of communication between early childhood professionals and the infants/children/families they serve. (The term "client" will be used to indicate the infant/child/family unit.) Letters, brochures, instructional handouts, reports and summaries, and Individualized Family Service Plans (IFSP) are examples of written materials used in the course of providing services to clients. For those who lack the reading skills necessary to understand such materials, however, it is only "so much paper"; they must rely on verbal explanations.

Current federal legislation has identified as a prime focus for professionals the enabling and empowering of families to better make their own choices and ultimately to meet their own needs. This often includes the provision of written materials pertinent to a topic of concern, or written instructions or ideas for parents and children to follow or explore. When extensive one-to-one counseling is precluded, instructional pamphlets and/or copies of magazine articles can be invaluable to both parents and professionals. Generally, it is expected that the clients share responsibility for progressing toward their goals, and that they will read, learn, and act upon the information provided. It is also assumed that comprehension is automatic. However, the reality is that simple receipt of information fails to translate directly into client understanding or behavioral change.

There are a number of ways for sensitive early childhood professionals (and others) to ease this situation and help those with low literacy skills to benefit from written materials. It takes only an awareness of what is possible, and perhaps a slight shift in the manner by which written information is provided.[1]

READABILITY OF MEDICAL INFORMATION

Accessibility of written information to clients is perhaps most crucial in the area of health care. Research in the health, mental health, or allied professions focusing on client comprehension of written materials is scant. Samora[2] and Larribee[3] found wide discrepancies in health care clients' understanding of medical vocabulary used to communicate with them. Mohammed,[4] in a study of patients in a diabetes clinic, found that 77% were unable to utilize the written information commonly provided at that time.

A sample of 291 widely used health instructions (many used nationally) was evaluated for reading level. The range of reading level was from 4th to 16th grade,

Inf Young Children 1991; 4(1): 62–67

with the mean at the 10th grade level.[1] Given that an estimated 50% of adult Americans read at the 8th to 9th grade level or below,[5] virtually none of these materials are likely to be comprehensible to individuals with low literacy skills, and even those with average skills will have some difficulty understanding them.[6] It therefore seems logical to deduce that an individual will have difficulty following instructions that are not understood. Failure to follow instructions provided only in written form may be viewed as evidence of a client's "bad attitude" and taken as simple noncompliance. A closer look at the process is warranted.

One way to take a closer look is to evaluate written materials in use for reading level. A number of formulae to test readability have been developed. They take into consideration the number of words and sentences, and the difficulty of the vocabulary in a sample passage. Difficulty of words is usually related to the number of syllables.[1,6] None of these formulae address factors such as the reader's level of knowledge or interest, or motivation for reading about a particular subject. They also do not evaluate the quality of writing.[2] Nevertheless, testing readability is a useful means of screening existing materials and can assist professionals in rewriting their materials for those functioning at lower reading levels.

One of the most accessible formulas for assessing reading level is the SMOG formula.[7] It is simple to use and can be done quickly. This method will determine the grade level of a sample passage to within 1½ grades 68% of the time.[6]

1. This test requires 30 sentences. A sentence is defined as any string of words punctuated by a period, exclamation point, or question mark. If a long sentence has a colon, consider each part as a separate sentence. Identify 10 consecutive sentences at the beginning, 10 from the middle, and 10 at the end. (By sampling each of these three locations you will get a more reliable idea of the overall reading level required.)

2. From the 30 sentences, count the number of words with 3 or more syllables. Include all repetitions. Numerals and abbreviations should be pronounced aloud to count syllables (eg, 250 equals 5 syllables; Dec. equals 3 syllables). Proper nouns should be included, and hyphenated words are considered 1 word. (For example, the sentence "Help Johnny to choose the clothes he will wear to school tomorrow each night before he goes to bed" would have a score of 1 because only 1 word, "tomorrow," has 3 or more syllables.)

3. Grade level may be calculated as follows: find the nearest perfect square root for the word count, then add a constant of 3 to that figure to find the grade level.[7]

For samples with fewer than 30 sentences:

1. Count the total number of sentences, then the number of multisyllable words.
2. Using Table 1, find the number of sentences and locate the conversion number in the opposite column.

Table 1. SMOG conversion for samples with fewer than 30 sentences

Number of sentences in sample material	*Conversion number*
29	1.03
28	1.07
27	1.1
26	1.15
25	1.2
24	1.25
23	1.3
22	1.36
21	1.43
20	1.5
19	1.58
18	1.67
17	1.76
16	1.87
15	2.0
14	2.14
13	2.3
12	2.5
11	2.7
10	3

Reprinted with permission from Doak CC, Doak LG, Root JH. *Teaching Patients with Low Literacy Skills.* Philadelphia, Pa: Lippincott; 1985.

3. Multiply the word count by the conversion number to obtain an adjusted word count. Proceed by finding the nearest perfect square root of the adjusted word count and add a constant of 3 to that figure to find the grade level.[1]

The SMOG formula can be helpful in comparing the difficulty of written material with suspected client ability. However, operationally defining "appropriate reading level" may be problematic. If material is written at too high a level, you may be courting mutual frustration with incomprehensible reading material. Yet, a common concern is that information written at a low level will be considered too basic[1] and either perceived by clients as insulting or simply dismissed outright. All we can do is strive to achieve the best match possible.

WRITING AND REWRITING

Whether rewriting existing materials or developing new materials, careful planning is essential. As you think about your project, consider: What, specifically, are your objectives (what is your purpose) for this piece of written material? What is it that you want your reader to know or do? What new knowledge will be learned? In identifying your objectives, many people find it helpful to frame them in concrete, testable outcomes (for example: "The reader will describe the planning steps that will simplify the task of writing."). Where appropriate, a criterion for measuring success can be included[1] (". . . will describe three planning steps. . .").

Identify the essential information you wish to convey, that information crucial to meeting your objectives. Extraneous information that you may find fascinating may simply be confusing to those not skilled in managing written information. The information must then be organized in a logical, straightforward manner. This is easy with progressive, step-wise instructions. In less obvious instances, material presented either first—or last—tends to be the most easily remembered. If several topics have equal importance, the one covering more general information should be presented first, followed by the next most specific.[1]

With the key points in mind and a sense of order about their presentation, you are ready to write. Keep in mind, however, that readability involves more than simply limiting the number of hard words or the length of text. One cardinal rule to be followed is to "write in an active voice in a conversational style."[6,8] In other words, use plain English, write the way you speak, and keep it simple. A message written in the active voice is more easily understood. Using the personal "you should . . ." in place of the abstract "the parent should . . ." has a greater impact[1] and so is often more effective for our purposes. Use simple words and sentences, making sure your text sounds natural. Naturalness is essential for ease of understanding.

Using simpler words is not talking down to your client; rather, by using his or her language, one conveys respect for the reader. As you write, read aloud what you have written. The text should flow naturally and easily, and progress in a logical manner. When in doubt, it is better to choose naturalness over "proper grammar" if it will help to achieve your goals.[8]

Be consistent in your use of terms. Rather than interchanging terms for the sake of variety, be consistent for the sake of clarity. For example, using "doctor," "physician," and then "health care provider" or "primary care physician" when referring to one individual may be colorful but can also be confusing. It is best to keep it simple and select the most familiar terms.[8]

Jargon should be avoided. While there are many ideas about what actually constitutes jargon, one rule of thumb is to consider whether a term has meaning to anyone who does not work regularly in your field. For example, the words "cognitive development" are considered basic terminology by most early childhood professionals; however, most of the general public can make better use of the phrase "thinking skills." Professional jargon does not convey information to the uninitiated, regardless of their reading skills. Where it is unavoidable, as when the simplest term is a jargon term, provide a clear definition with the first use of the word in the text.[8]

Organize the text in a way that will help the reader focus on what is to follow and enhance ease of understanding. Headings can be used as advance organizers. This provides important cues about the intended message. It is best to limit each paragraph to its main topic and supporting facts. Multiple messages in one paragraph will muddy the waters.[8] By keeping one idea per paragraph, written material is more generally accessible.

That old homily for lecture preparation, "Tell them what you're going to tell them, tell them, then tell them what you've told them" can also be applied to writing. Summary and review sections are important. Present the information again in a new format, such as a question and answer section, or a self-assessment quiz at the end of the piece.[1]

In summary, remember: As you are reading this text, you are taking in whole ideas, reading groups of words. Those with low literacy skills tend to see each word individually and decode it one letter at a time, every time it is encountered; only then can they begin to decipher the ideas being presented. This is a monumental task. Strive for simplicity, clarity, and naturalness. Organize information logically, offering only that which is essential for understanding. Choose familiar terms and be consistent. Avoid jargon whenever possible. Remember too that the average number of new ideas a person is able to grasp and retain is around seven.[1] Consequently, keep the concept density (or number of ideas presented in a passage or paragraph) low. You don't want the major message to get lost in extraneous information. Summarize and review. And, if you remember nothing else, remember this: "When writing for low reading levels, use a conversational style and the active voice."[1(p74)]

PRESENTATION OF WRITTEN MATERIALS

When you have completed the text, take some time to consider the format of the final product. Some items of concern are print size and type style, line width, and use of color. Many of these considerations can be discussed with your printer.

A simple type style should be selected. The use of both upper and lower case type is best, as the humps and bumps and the above- and below-line characteristics of letters can aid in letter and word recognition. A text written with all capitals or upper case letters presents a more uniform image and so may be more difficult to read. Script type or italics are also more difficult to decipher. For these reasons, <u>underline</u> words in order to add emphasis rather than using capitals or italics. Symbols should be written out and abbreviations avoided (ie, use "add" for "+", "equals" for "=", and "October" for "Oct.").[6] Doak et al[1] recommend a larger type size, specifically, 14-point type (Fig 1 illustrates type sizes).

The selection of ink and paper color should be based on the degree of contrast between them. In general, a sharp contrast assists the readers' perception and com-

This is a sample of the 8 point type.

This is a sample of the 10 point type.

This is a sample of the 12 point type.

This is a sample of the 14 point type.

This is a sample of the 18 point type.

Fig 1. Common type sizes. Reprinted with permission from Doak CC, Doak LG, Root JH. *Teaching Patients with Low Literacy Skills.* Philadelphia, Pa: Lippincott; 1985.

---

prehension. Black or dark print on a white or light yellow background tend to be good choices; be wary of the medium or darker shades of pink, blue, or green.[9]

A shorter line width, as when text is printed in two columns on a page, tends to aid understanding. This format requires a shorter scanning field and results in longer eye fixation on the text.[10]

TEACHING WITH WRITTEN MATERIALS

Some early childhood professionals may question their role and ability as teachers of reading skills to the parents of their clients; there are, however, many opportunities to assist families with this essential dimension of life *while in the process* of meeting the child's goals and needs.

Providing written materials, even to those who cannot read well, should be seen as an opportunity for the parent that is very much related to the welfare of the child (if not the whole family). Take the opportunity to model ways one can use written information for help and reassurance. It is important to discuss with the parent what the written material "says" and then leave it for them to review. Your common goals in providing the material may serve as motivation for many parents to seek additional help with their literacy skills.

When discussing written information, it is important to seek feedback from your clients to evaluate their understanding of what was said. Keeping in mind the tendency to conceal low literacy skills, you won't get far if you simply ask "Do you understand?" Ask specific questions, or ask the client to solve a sample problem. Another method is to ask the client to tell you in his or her own words what was described, or have the client explain the information to another family member[6] in your presence.

Since you are the early childhood professional, the "expert," practically any interaction with the client can be considered a teaching episode. The ripples of your interest and efforts on behalf of others can spread in unforeseen directions. A small amount of time devoted to assisting parents with literacy skills may literally turn the world around for them. In the interests of the children, this falls well within our scope of early childhood intervention.

REFERENCES

1. Doak C, Doak LG, Root JH. *Teaching Patients with Low Literacy Skills.* Philadelphia, Pa: Lippincott; 1985.
2. Samora J. Medical vocabulary knowledge among hospital patients. *J Health Hum Behav.* 1961;2(2):83–90.
3. Larribee PD. *Patient understanding of vocabulary terms used in initial health assessment.* Rochester, NY: Univ Rochester; 1977. Dissertation.
4. Mohammed M. Patient understanding of written health information. *Nurs Res.* 1964;13:108.
5. Adult Performance Level Project. *Final Report: The APL Study.* Austin, Tex: The APL Project; 1978.
6. Costa Marie. *Adult Literacy/Illiteracy in the United States.* Santa Barbara, Calif: ABC-CLIO; 1988.
7. McLaughlin GH. SMOG Grading—A new readability formula. *Journal of Reading.* 1969;12:639–646.
8. Flesch RF. *The Art of Readable Writing.* New York, NY: Collier Books; 1962.
9. Paterson DG, Tinker MA. Studies of typographical factors influencing speed of reading. *J Appl Psychol.* 1941;15:241–247.
10. Paterson DG, Tinker MA. Influences of line width on eye movement. *J Exp Psychol,* 1940;27:572–577.

Acoustic amplification for hearing-impaired infants and young children

Jackson Roush, PhD
Assistant Professor
Division of Speech and Hearing Sciences
University of North Carolina Medical School
Chapel Hill, North Carolina

THE DEVELOPMENT of the auditory mechanism and the onset of hearing normally begin several months prior to birth. By the 20th week of gestation, the inner ear reaches adult size and differentiation, the only sensory organ to do so in utero.[1] Middle and external ear structures, although not of adult size, are well formed by the 30th gestational week. Soon after birth, the neonate exhibits a variety of impressive auditory behaviors, including sound localization[2] and frequency/intensity discriminations.[3] Even more impressive is the infant's ability to identify phonemic contrasts, linguistic stress, and other precursors of speech and language development.[4]

Considering the complexities of normal auditory development, it is not surprising that a hearing loss of early onset has serious implications for speech and language development. Even a mild hearing loss can cause delays in speech and language, and more severe losses invariably have a profound impact on the development of expressive as well as receptive verbal communication.[5] Fortunately, techniques for the identification of hearing loss have improved substantially making it possible to consider acoustic amplification at a very early age. The majority of hearing-impaired children derive substantial benefit from some form of acoustic amplification,[6] especially when it is initiated early and maintained consistently.[7,8]

The purpose of this article is to examine the various options available for acoustic amplification in hearing-impaired infants and toddlers. Primary emphasis will be given to the management of amplification in children with hearing losses of a permanent (sensorineural) type. Controversial and unresolved issues will be addressed as well as a number of important interdisciplinary concerns related to this population.

IDENTIFICATION OF HEARING LOSS AND MEASUREMENT OF HEARING

It is estimated that approximately 1 of every 750 infants in the well-baby population will be born with a bilateral sensorineural hearing impairment of some de-

This work was sponsored in part by a grant from the US Department of Maternal and Child Health as part of a collaborative project with The Carolina Institute for Research on Infant Personnel Preparation at the University of North Carolina, Chapel Hill.
The author thanks Bruce Weber, Barbara Herrmann, Jerry Northern, and two anonymous reviewers for their constructive comments on an earlier version of this article.

Inf Young Children 1990; 2(4): 59–71

gree.[9] When infants at high risk (eg, neonatal intensive care unit [NICU] graduates) are considered separately, the incidence increases dramatically, to approximately 1 of 25 to 50.[10,11] As a result, it is now common practice in many medical centers to screen for hearing loss in the high-risk population. In a recent issue of *Infants and Young Children,* Cox[12] discussed the advantages and disadvantages of various screening procedures. On the basis of a review of published research, he recommends that children who are at risk for hearing loss, as well as all NICU graduates, regardless of whether they qualify for the high-risk register, be evaluated electrophysiologically by auditory brainstem response (ABR) test procedures. Although behavioral test procedures may appear to be more convenient and cost-effective, the overall predictive accuracy of ABR makes it the test of choice for the identification of hearing loss in high-risk neonates. For older infants, behavioral test procedures, including visual reinforcement audiometry (VRA), are useful in the assessment of aided as well as unaided response levels. Briefly, VRA is conducted using calibrated auditory signals presented from a loudspeaker in a sound-treated room. When the infant turns toward the sound source, reinforcement is provided by an attractive visual display, usually consisting of a light and a moving toy. The procedure is useful in establishing minimum auditory response levels in normally developing youngsters from 6 months to 2 years of age.[13] (For more details on behavioral and electrophysiologic testing in young children, refer to the recent articles in *Infants and Young Children* by Cox[12] and Madell.[14])

The advent of ABR as a screening tool has greatly improved the accuracy and timeliness of the initial identification. ABR is also useful with older children, particularly those with multiple handicaps. Behavioral tests such as VRA are useful in infants whose developmental age is 6 months and beyond. Planning for initial aural habilitation is best accomplished with a combination of behavioral and electrophysiologic test procedures.

OPTIONS FOR ACOUSTIC AMPLIFICATION

Hearing aids come in a variety of styles and sizes ranging from large body-worn instruments to devices small enough to be concealed in the ear canal. Despite this array of fitting options, certain characteristics are common to all acoustic amplification devices. As illustrated in Fig 1, all hearing aids have a microphone, an amplifier, a receiver, and a volume control. In addition, most have external controls to adjust the frequency response and maximum output. A battery, usually a disposable mercury or zinc air cell, is also required.

For infants and toddlers, the most practical options are generally the body-worn and behind-the-ear instruments (see Fig 2, a and b). The larger body-worn aids are often selected for very young children because the greater separation between microphone and receiver reduces problems associated with acoustic feedback.

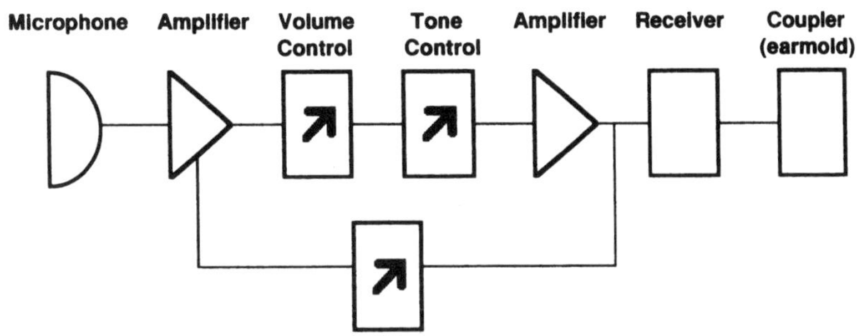

Fig 1. Block diagram showing the basic components of a typical hearing aid.

Acoustic feedback is familiar to anyone who has ever used a public address system: when the microphone comes into proximity with the loudspeaker, a disturbing squeal persists until the two devices are moved farther apart or a barrier is created between them. In the context of the hearing aid, the barrier is created by a custom-made earmold (Fig 3) that helps to secure the instrument to the ear while providing an acoustic seal. Even when the earmold is tightly fitted, however, problems with acoustic feedback may necessitate the use of a body-worn aid to increase the distance between the microphone and receiver. For young children with mild to moderate hearing losses, it is usually possible to begin with ear-level amplification; for others, the body-worn hearing aid is a temporary fitting until ear-level amplification is feasible. Advantages of an ear-level fitting include the elimination of clothing noise, easier maintenance, better appearance, and improved binaural (two-eared) hearing, since the microphones can be located at ear level. The potential advantages of an ear-level fitting, however, are of little consequence if acoustic feedback prevents the instruments from delivering the amplification needs. For young children with severe to profound hearing losses, body-worn hearing aids are capable of providing consistent, high-quality amplification, even at high output levels. In addition, the placement of the microphones on the chest enables the body to serve as a baffle, which results in an enhancement of the hearing aid's low-frequency response.[15] When two separate hearing aids are fitted, as illustrated in Fig 2a, true binaural stimulation can be achieved with body-worn instruments.

Another important option for acoustic amplification in children is the radio frequency (FM) system. Such a fitting is shown in Fig 4, which illustrates the use of binaural ear-level instruments in conjunction with an FM transmitter and receiver. Since this type of instrument employs an external microphone, FM transmissions can provide selective amplification of the primary sound source (the speech of the parent or teacher wearing the FM transmitter) with less interference from back-

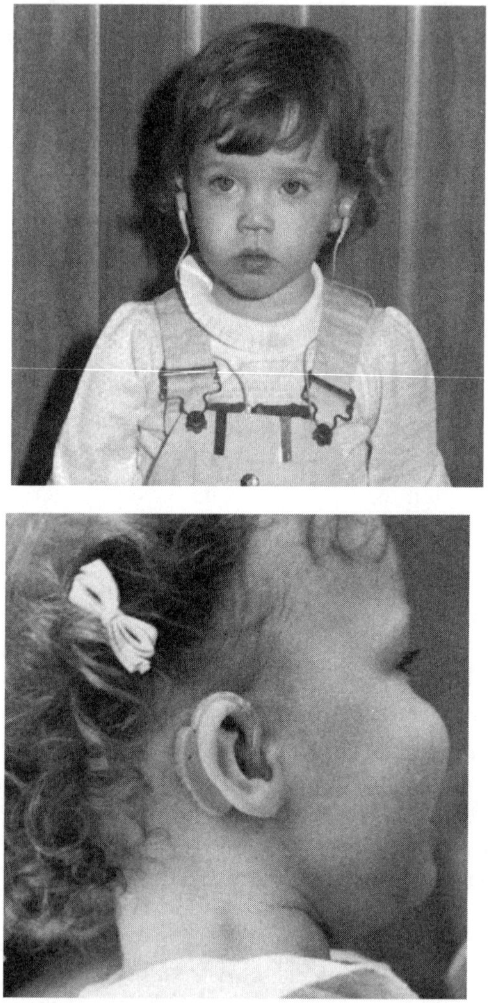

Fig 2. (**a**) Body-worn and (**b**) behind-the-ear hearing aids are the types most commonly used with infants and young children.

ground noise. Since the FM system can transmit and receive signals over a considerable distance, the device can also improve the quality of amplification when the child is not nearby. When the FM transmitter is turned off, the device can be worn as a standard hearing aid. Used in that manner, the instrument employs two separate microphones and receivers, which allows the listener to enjoy the benefit of binaural stimulation without two separate body-worn instruments. Although the

a

b

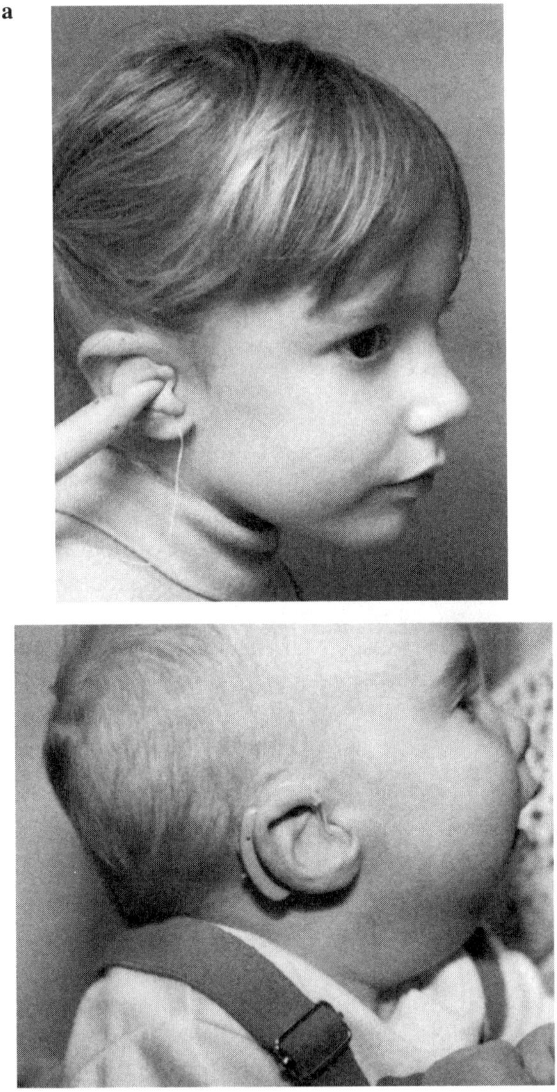

Fig 3. (**a**) An ear impression is used by an earmold laboratory to fabricate (**b**) a custom earmold. When used with a behind-the-ear hearing aid like the one shown here, the earmold is attached to the hearing aid by a short length of flexible tubing.

device is slightly larger than a standard body-worn hearing aid, it can often be used successfully, even with infants and toddlers. Because of its electroacoustic flexibility, its ability to provide high-quality amplification in a variety of listening

a

b

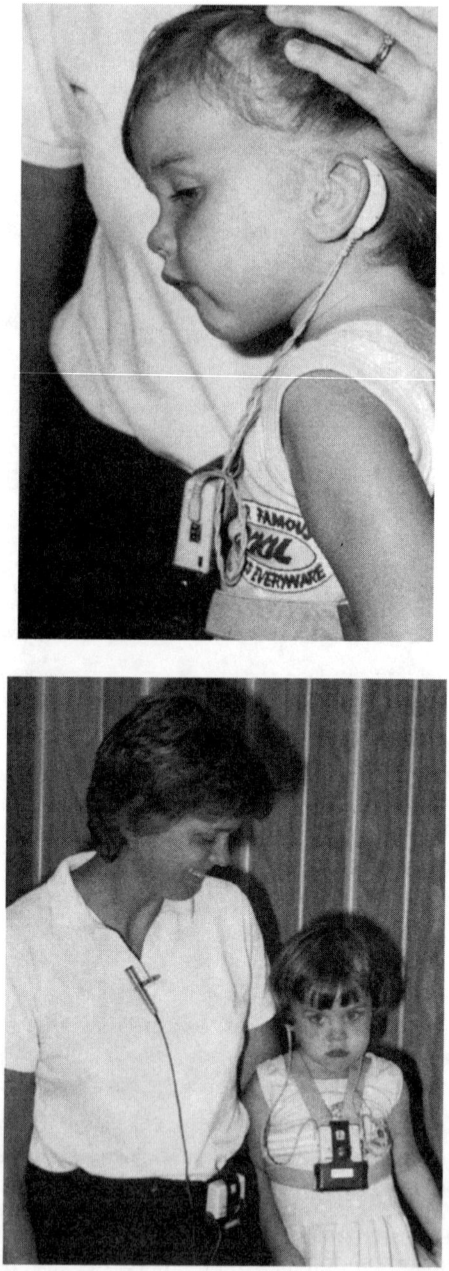

Fig 4. (**a**) This FM system uses ear-level hearing aids in conjuntion with an FM receiver worn on the body. (**b**) The child's mother is shown wearing an FM transmitter.

conditions, and its capability of delivering high output levels with minimal interference from acoustic feedback, the FM instrument is becoming increasingly popular for use by hearing-impaired infants and toddlers.

EVALUATION OF ACOUSTIC AMPLIFICATION

Once hearing aids are selected and fitted, an evaluation of aided performance is needed to assess the benefits obtained. For adults and older children, it is possible to use standardized materials consisting of various speech stimuli that the listener is asked to repeat. To evaluate their ability to tolerate extremely loud sounds, adults and older children can be asked to report their subjective judgments of discomfort as progressively louder sounds are presented. Such procedures are not feasible with infants and young children, although behavioral observation and visual reinforcement audiometry can be used in conjunction with speech and tonal stimuli to compare aided and unaided response levels. Judgments of loudness discomfort are more difficult because of the considerable variability in children's behavioral responses to high intensity stimulation.

Recently, a new clinical assessment procedure has emerged that offers potentially greater control over the initial selection of response characteristics in hearing aids for young hearing-impaired children. Known as "real ear probe microphone measurements," these procedures permit an objective assessment of the hearing aid's amplification characteristics as measured under actual listening conditions. Because there are significant differences in the ear's size, shape, canal volume, and impedance characteristics from one person to another, real ear measures obtained via probe microphone technology are useful in specifying the actual sound pressure levels existing in the ear canal of the listener.

In Fig 5, probe microphone measurements are being obtained in the ear of a 4-month-old infant. An initial measurement is made by placing the flexible probe tube into the unaided ear canal. This tube leads to a microphone and a measuring device that provides a graphic display of the real ear amplification characteristics. The unaided measurement is used to determine the resonance and other external ear effects in the ear canal *without* amplification. The hearing aid, attached to a custom-made earmold, is then inserted over the probe tube, and an *aided* measurement is obtained. The difference between the aided and unaided levels can be calculated to determine the insertion gain, or the amount of amplification added by the hearing aid when it is fitted to the ear. To examine the hearing aid's maximum amplification level in the ear, the stimulus can be increased until the hearing aid reaches saturation, the point at which further amplification ceases to occur even when the input levels are increased.

Measurements of insertion gain and maximum output are critical to the successful fitting of amplification in young children. Overamplification will cause some children to reject hearing aid use, and in some, it can be damaging to the ear, even

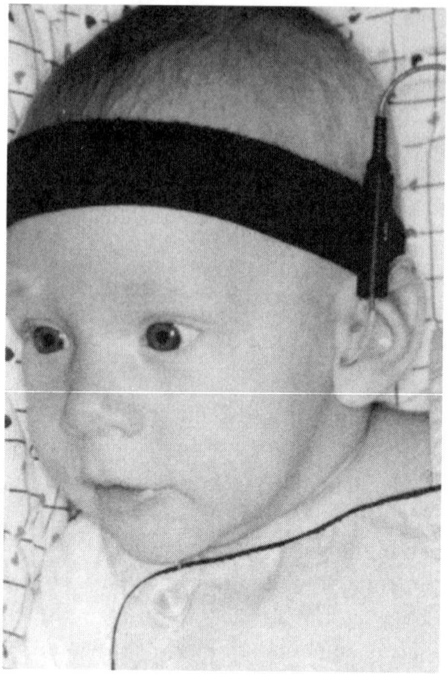

Fig 5. Probe microphone techniques permit direct measurement of the amplified sound pressure levels in the ear canal. To obtain these measurements, a small probe tube is placed in the ear canal and the earmold is inserted over it.

in the absence of any overt behavioral evidence. Conversely, an overly conservative approach leading to underamplification can result in levels too low to provide sufficient auditory stimulation. Considering the relatively small volume of the ear canal in young children, output levels tend to be higher than one would expect from the hearing aid manufacturer's technical description of the instrument. The manufacturer's specifications are based on measurements obtained with the hearing aid attached to a standard coupler in a calibrated test chamber (Fig 6). Electroacoustic measurements obtained in this manner are useful for monitoring the functional status of a hearing aid or determining whether it conforms to technical specifications, but the resulting output is likely to differ significantly from the response in the real ear, especially in children.[16] Because sound levels tend to increase as the ear canal volume decreases, hearing-impaired infants may be inadvertently "over-fitted" unless appropriate allowances are made. As probe microphone instrumentation becomes more widely available and used with young children, the likelihood of such errors will be greatly diminished.

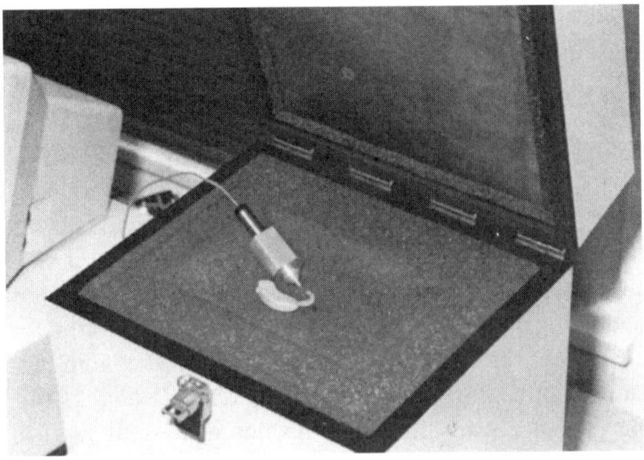

Fig 6. For standard electroacoustic measurements, the hearing aid is attached to a 2-cc coupler and placed in an acoustic test chamber.

It is important to note that probe microphone measurements, although useful in determining actual sound pressure levels in the ear canal, cannot specify the electroacoustic characteristics that are truly optimal for a given individual. Furthermore, they cannot provide an indication of what the child actually perceives. They can, however, guide the audiologist in the selection of a safe and appropriate initial fitting, which can be modified, as needed, over time. When the child is older, it is usually possible to obtain direct measurements of aided performance by using speech stimuli in conjunction with behavioral test procedures.

Regardless of the specific evaluation procedures employed, the goal in pediatric hearing aid selection is to provide an amplified speech signal that will give access to the widest possible frequency range, at intensity levels that are within the child's tolerance.[17] As such, the hearing aid does not correct the hearing impairment; rather, it increases the intensity of speech so that the impaired ear can have access to the acoustic information that it is able to perceive.

In addition to a loss of hearing sensitivity, the impaired auditory system causes distortion of incoming signals. The level of this inherent distortion tends to increase with the degree of hearing loss, making conventional amplification of limited value in cases of profound impairment. Nevertheless, acoustic amplification can be used effectively in the vast majority of hearing-impaired children, even when there is minimal residual hearing.[7] It is important to recognize, however, that, regardless of the degree of hearing impairment, hearing aid use does not restore "normal hearing" even when amplification is appropriately selected and fitted.

Most permanent hearing losses in children are due to abnormal inner ear function, that is, sensorineural impairment. However, congenital conditions characterized by middle and external ear anomalies (Fig 7a) are often associated with normal inner ear function, resulting in a conductive impairment. When the use of a standard earmold and hearing aid is not feasible and the inner ear function is normal, a bone conduction hearing aid may be indicated. When sound is converted to a vibrotactile stimulus, the amplified signal can be conveyed directly to the inner ear by a bone vibrator worn on the head. In Fig 7b, an infant is shown wearing a bone conduction transducer attached to a metal headband. With infants and young children, such fittings are often more practical if the bone vibrator is contained within a small pocket fitted to an elastic headband, as shown in Fig 7c. Although somewhat cumbersome, this arrangement can provide useful amplification to aid in speech and language acquisition and development, until surgical intervention can be undertaken to resolve the conductive impairment. For those few who are not surgical candidates, an implantable version of this device has been developed recently.[18] Its usefulness with children, however, is still being evaluated.

CONTROVERSIAL AND UNRESOLVED ISSUES

Hearing aid selection based on ABR

It is generally agreed that acoustic amplification should be provided as soon as possible after a hearing impairment is discovered. There is some disagreement, however, as to whether electrophysiologic test results are sufficient to confirm the nature and degree of a hearing impairment or whether the hearing aid fitting should be deferred until corroborating behavioral test data can be obtained. This practice can delay the fitting of amplification for several months, and even longer for some children with multiple handicaps.

There are two general areas of concern regarding the validity of ABR as a test of hearing sensitivity. First, it has been shown that a variety of transient neurologic disorders can create abnormal and, in some cases, reversible ABR patterns.[19] For example, premature infants, particularly those with a history of acute asphyxia, may demonstrate severe ABR abnormalities,[20] even when hearing sensitivity is normal. Fortunately, such findings are rare and can sometimes be identified by the experienced ABR clinician for more conservative audiologic follow-up. Second, it is sometimes difficult to define the nature of the hearing loss with respect to the child's hearing sensitivity across the frequency range. The stimulus most commonly used in ABR evaluations, an acoustic "click," provides information only in the range of 1000 to 4000 Hz. Glattke[21] showed that this stimulus will yield ABR patterns that are similar regardless of low-frequency hearing status. Obviously the amplification needs of a child with normal low-frequency hearing are quite different from those of a child with equal hearing loss in the low and high frequencies. A

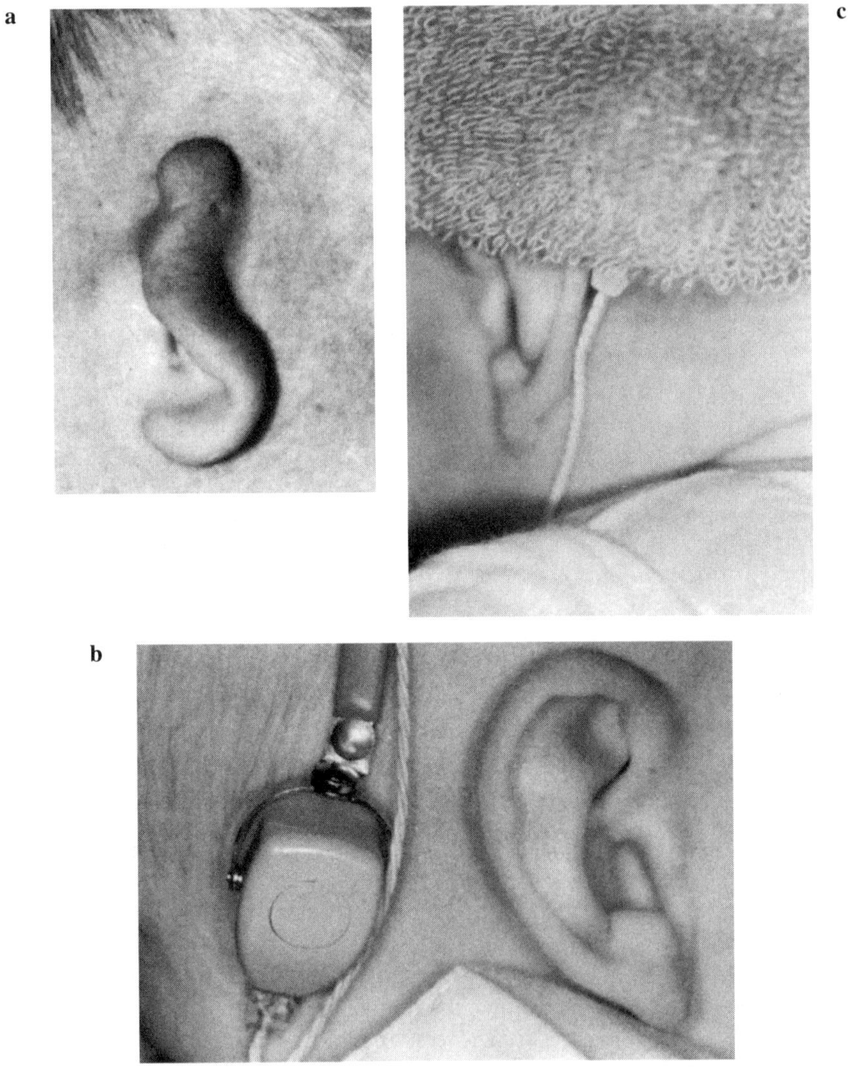

Fig 7. (**a**) Congenital malformation of the external ear and other conditions may preclude the use of a standard earmold and hearing aid. In such cases, inner ear function is often normal, and a conductive hearing loss can be overcome by means of a bone vibrator attached to (**b**) a steel spring or (**c**) an elastic headband.

variety of techniques for achieving improved frequency specificity have been described in the audiologic literature,[22,23] and it is often possible to use toneburst stimuli with different test parameters to reliably obtain a frequency-specific estimate that can be useful for planning aural habilitation.[24] Such procedures require skilled examiners, however, who are aware of the potential pitfalls as well as the benefits of these techniques.[25]

Problems related to frequency-specificity are also encountered when attempts are made to use the ABR for comparison of evoked potentials obtained with and without amplification (ie, to use ABR as a means of conducting an objective hearing aid evaluation). Specifically, click-evoked ABRs usually fail to differentiate hearing aids with varying degrees of low-frequency amplification.[26] Attempts to use the ABR in this manner have been further complicated by electromagnetic artifacts from the hearing aid that tend to alter the frequency response and temporal characteristics.[27] For a review of the potential benefits and limitations of ABR in the selection and evaluation of hearing aids for young children, the interested reader is referred to Beauchaine and Gorga.[27]

It is clear that ABR is an essential part of the pediatric test protocol, but it must be applied judiciously when used in planning aural habilitation for young children. With more effective use of existing ABR techniques, the delay from identification to intervention should be substantially reduced. Future developments in auditory electrophysiology will undoubtedly lead to even better techniques for identifying the nature and degree of a hearing loss as well as the effects of acoustic amplification.

Binaural hearing aids

Although once controversial, binaural fitting is now widely accepted as appropriate and desirable in nearly all cases of bilateral sensorineural hearing loss, especially in children. Despite this apparent consensus, however, many children are still fitted monaurally who could benefit from binaural stimulation.[28] As previously stated, true binaural amplification requires the use of a separate microphone and receiver for each ear. Assuming that there is residual hearing in both ears, binaural amplification can be easily accomplished with two individual behind-the-ear hearing aids. When body-worn instruments are required, it is still possible to achieve a binaural fitting (Fig 2b), although the arrangement is more cumbersome. In either case, binaural amplification is essential for enhanced sound localization and improved speech perception in adverse listening conditions. If, as suggested by Ross,[29] a delay in providing two hearing aids can result in less optimal binaural performance later on, it seems best to attempt a binaural fitting as soon as practical, whether the initial fitting is with body-worn or ear-level hearing aids.

Parental acceptance

The issue of ear-level *v* body-worn amplification was considered earlier from a technical standpoint. An equally important concern, however, is that of parental perception and willingness to accept a more unsightly and obtrusive hardware arrangement in favor of improved amplification for the child. Although research in this area is lacking, it is possible that the hearing aids may, in some cases, interfere with the process of parent–child bonding. In most cases, however, parents will be most accepting of the amplification arrangement that provides the greatest overall benefit, regardless of physical appearance. Matkin[30] points out that a hearing loss is an invisible handicap until the hearing aids are introduced. Clinicians should be sensitive to this and take the time needed to explain the goals, benefits, and rationale for a given hearing-aid fitting, in a manner that is understandable and meaningful to parents and family members.

The issue of parental acceptance has significance beyond the selection of the hearing instrument per se. Luterman[31] notes that professionals involved with young hearing-impaired children often interpret resistance or noncompliance on matters of hearing aid use as evidence of parental negligence, and they respond by offering admonitions that serve only to further increase the parents' sense of inadequacy. Instead, Luterman advises clinicians to recognize these behaviors as normal psychological reactions to a situation that, for most parents, is a strange and frightening one. A supportive, nonjudgmental environment will enable most parents to work through these emotions and eventually to participate constructively in planning the habilitation program.[32]

Alternatives to acoustic amplification

Sometimes conventional hearing aids are found to provide little or no benefit. For those few individuals with hearing losses too severe to benefit from acoustic amplification, a cochlear implant or a vibrotactile aid may be recommended.

Briefly, a cochlear implant consists of a series of electrodes placed in the inner ear and attached to an induction coil buried under the skin near the ear. From an external device, amplified signals are then delivered to the internal coil and conveyed to the electrodes, which provide direct simulation to the auditory nerve. Consideration of a cochlear implant is appropriate only after it has been determined that conventional amplification is of no practical benefit. There is considerable controversy, however, regarding how and when this decision is made. To date, the best pediatric candidates for cochlear implants have been children with *acquired* hearing losses, that is, those who experienced normal speech–language development for a period of time. A strong auditory–oral approach to early intervention is also likely to improve the prognosis for success with an implant regardless of etiology. Many unanswered questions remain concerning patient selection, implant design, and optimal processing strategies, but it seems likely that cochlear implants will continue to improve, and thus offer potentially greater benefits in the future. For further information on cochlear implants in children, the interested reader is referred to Owens and Kessler.[33]

Vibrotactile devices present amplified speech signals through vibrating stimulators worn on the forearm, forehead, or sternum. There are also "electrocutaneous" devices that present speech signals as electrical pulses to the skin.[34] Although these devices are, because of their noninvasive nature, less controversial than cochlear implants, they have had limited application with young children. In recent years, however, technologic advances have greatly improved their benefit and wearability. As a result, more widespread pediatric application of these devices is expected in the future. A review of these and other nontraditional sensory aids for the hearing-impaired was recently published by the *Volta Review*.[35]

Delays in intervention and follow-up

A matter of continuing concern is that of follow-up, both in terms of the initial fitting and with respect to ongoing management. Despite universal agreement regarding the virtues of early intervention, there are still, in many cases, inordinate delays in completing the initial fitting of amplification after a hearing loss has been discovered. Most parents report that their initial expressions of concern to a pediatrician or family physician were not taken seriously, and, as a result, the identification process was delayed for several months. Even after the hearing loss is discovered, there are often further delays. In 1980, Simmons[36] examined the records of 42 hearing-impaired children whose average age at the initial hearing aid fitting was 22 months. His review revealed that 83% were suspected of having a hearing loss prior to their discharge from the newborn nursery, and of those who were not suspect at the time of discharge, nearly half failed an initial hearing test prior to the age of 1 year. In a discussion of these data, Northern and Downs[1] note that the typical delays between identification and fitting fall into one of three patterns:

1. a long, silent interval of no action following referral back to the child's physician,
2. the manifestation by a child with multiple handicaps, of which hearing is only one, and
3. parental disbelief regarding the diagnosis of hearing impairment.

Although such patterns are not entirely avoidable, a dedication to comprehensive and individualized family counseling and a commitment to interdisciplinary cooperation can expedite the process of early intervention.

Equally important is the provision of regular audiologic follow-up after habilitation has been initiated. Too often, the flurry of activity surrounding an initial hearing aid fitting is followed by sporadic and incomplete monitoring of the child's hearing status and the status of the hearing instruments. Considering the importance of acoustic amplification and its many potential complications, hearing-impaired preschoolers should be monitored audiologically at least every 4 to 6 months, even when there are no apparent changes. When follow-up is a problem, early interventionists involved with the family on a regular basis can assist by ensuring that ongoing audiologic monitoring is consistently provided.

Finally, the child and family will need access to a comprehensive program of guidance, counseling, and educational support that is appropriate to their needs.[37] Such programs range from family-centered models aimed at enabling parents to become co-therapists[38] to programs that are essentially child-centered in nature. Because there is tremendous variability in cultural, socioeconomic, and family systems, a variety of service delivery models must be provided whenever possible.[39] Unfortunately, many families with hearing-impaired infants and toddlers do not have access to early intervention services that are appropriate to their needs. The recent amendments to Public Law 99-457 are intended to improve the quality and availability of services to infants and toddlers with special needs and their families.

INTERDISCIPLINARY ISSUES

In most cases, sensorineural hearing loss in children cannot be treated medically, and the audiologist assumes responsibility for the first step in treatment and management: the selection and fitting of amplification. Once the hearing aid fitting has been completed, however, the child's habilitative management involves a variety of professionals, all of whom play an important part in maximizing the child's use of residual hearing. It is important to emphasize that the fitting of hearing aids is a continual process that is likely to change as the child develops and as observations from parents and professionals are considered. Since the audiologist is more likely to see the child in a clinical environment, family members and specialists from other disciplines are generally in the best position to observe the benefits of amplification in various listening situations. Moreover, it is the responsibility of those who see the child outside the audiologic setting to ensure that the hearing aids are worn, that the earmolds are properly inserted, that external controls are at the prescribed settings, and that batteries are functional and properly inserted. Regrettably, history has shown that these goals are not easily accomplished. The audiology literature is replete with surveys from the 1960s to the 1980s, showing that at any given time, approximately half the hearing aids being worn by hearing-impaired children were functioning inappropriately.[40] Only through effective parent or caretaker orientation and interdisciplinary cooperation can this unfortunate state of affairs be ameliorated. A dialogue among the audiologist, the family, and other professionals working with the family should be established to ensure proper orientation to the care and use of the hearing aids and to implement a mechanism for providing feedback to the audiologist regarding the child's progress with amplification. Children with multiple handicaps, in particular, require careful long-term observation to judge the benefits of amplification.

Of importance equal to the hearing aids themselves is a critical examination of the auditory environment in which amplification is used. It is well known that hearing-impaired individuals are more detrimentally affected by noise, reverberation, and other adverse listening conditions than are those with normal hearing.[41]

Even the best efforts to achieve optimal amplification and early intervention can be thwarted by a poor acoustic environment. The audiologist should consult with family members and professionals involved on a day-to-day basis to evaluate the listening environment and make whatever modifications are reasonable.

Finally, professionals from all disciplines need to participate in the identification of *undetected* hearing impairments. Delays in initial identification are not uncommon, particularly in infants and young children with multiple handicaps. Many communities do not have screening programs for infants at risk for hearing loss, and even where such programs exist, a hearing impairment may be present despite the absence of high-risk conditions. In fact, Stein et al[11] estimate that one third to one half of hearing-impaired children have no apparent high-risk factors for hearing loss. The possibility of an acquired or progressive hearing loss also should be considered. Professionals working with infants and young children with handicaps must be watchful for signs of hearing impairment and seek otologic and audiologic evaluation whenever the hearing status is questionable or appears to be changing.

When multiple disciplines are involved in early intervention with handicapped children and their families, well-coordinated professional communication is critical. But the management of acoustic amplification and the related intervention needed to facilitate optimal hearing requires a spirit of professional interaction that goes beyond the usual boundaries of interdisciplinary cooperation. Although some audiologists may be able to offer direct service in the child's home or day-care environment, this is not a realistic expectation for most. What is needed is a "transdisciplinary" model that, according to Bailey,[42] should be aimed at a blending of roles, enabling primary caregivers and other professionals to implement recommendations by practitioners from other disciplines. Such a model requires an open-minded attitude toward traditional roles and an appreciation for the long-term benefits of enabling others to share in those roles.

For most hearing-impaired children, acoustic amplification is the single most important component of early habilitation. Successful use of acoustic amplification requires the collaboration of professionals and family members to ensure the optimal use of each child's auditory capabilities.

REFERENCES

1. Northern J, Downs M. *Hearing in Children.* Baltimore: Williams & Wilkins; 1984.
2. Field J, Muir D, Pilon R, et al. Infant's orientation to lateral sounds from birth to three months. *Child Dev.* 1980; 51:295–298.
3. Eisenberg R. *Auditory Competence in Early Life.* Baltimore: University Park Press; 1976.

4. Kuhl P. Infant speech perception: Reviewing data on auditory category formation. In: Levinson P, Sloan C, eds. *Auditory Processing and Language: Clinical and Research Perspectives.* New York: Grune & Stratton; 1980.
5. Davis J, Hardick E. Language and speech characteristics. *Rehabilitative Audiology for Children and Adults.* New York: Wiley; 1981.
6. Erber N. Speech perception by hearing impaired children. In: Bess F, Friedman B, Sinclair J, eds. *Amplification in Education.* Washington, DC: A.G. Bell Association for the Deaf; 1981.
7. Ling D, Leckie D, Pollack D, et al. Syllable reception by hearing impaired children trained from infancy in auditory-oral programs. *Volta Rev.* 1981;83:451–457.
8. Markides A. Age of fitting of hearing aids and speech intelligibility. *Br. J Audiol.* 1986;20:165–167.
9. Downs M. The rationale for neonatal hearing screening. In: Sweigart E, ed. *Neonatal Hearing Screening.* San Diego: College Hill Press; 1986.
10. Cox LC, Hack M, Metz D. Auditory brainstem response audiometry in very low birth weight infants: incidence and risk factors. *Ear Hear.* 1984;5:47–51.
11. Stein L, Ozdamar O, Kraus N, et al. Follow-up of infants screened by auditory brainstem response in the neonatal intensive care unit. *J Pediatr.* 1983;103:447–453.
12. Cox LC. Screening the high-risk newborn for hearing loss: the Crib-O-Gram *v* the auditory brainstem response. *Inf Young Children.* 1988;(1):71–81.
13. Wilson W, Thompson G. Behavioral audiometry. In: Jerger J, ed. *Pediatric Audiology.* San Diego: College Hill Press; 1984.
14. Madell J. Identification and treatment of very young children with hearing loss. *Inf Young Children.* 1988;1(2):20–30.
15. Erber N. Body-baffle and real-ear effects in the selection of hearing aids for deaf children. *J Speech Hear Disord.* 1973;38:224–231.
16. Feigin J, Kopun J. Stelmachowicz P, et al. Probe microphone measurements of sound pressure levels in infants and children. Paper presented at the annual meeting of the American Speech-Language-Hearing Association, New Orleans, La, November 1987.
17. Seewald R, Ross M. Amplification for young hearing impaired children. In: Pollack M, ed. *Amplification for the Hearing Impaired.* Orlando, Fla: Grune & Stratton; 1988.
18. Hough J, Himelick T, Johnson B. Implantable bone conduction hearing device. *Ann Otol Rhinol Laryngol.* 1986;95:498–504.
19. Staller S. Auditory brain stem response and electrocochleography. In: Lass N, McReynolds L, Northern J, Yoder D, eds. *The Handbook of Speech-Language Pathology and Audiology.* Toronto: B.C. Decker; 1988.
20. Hecox K, Cone B. Prognostic importance of brainstem auditory evoked responses after asphyxia. *Neurology.* 1981;31:1429–1433.
21. Glattke T. *Short-Latency Auditory Evoked Potentials.* Austin, Tex: PRO-ED; 1983.
22. Kileny P, Magathan J. Predictive value of ABR in infants and children with moderate to profound hearing impairment. *Ear Hear.* 1987;8:217–221.
23. Gorga M, Kaminshi J, Beauchaine K. Auditory brainstem responses to high-frequency tone bursts in normal hearing subjects. *Ear Hear.* 1987;8:222–223.
24. Berlin C, Hood L. Auditory brainstem response and middle ear assessment in children. In: Martin F, ed. *Hearing Disorders in Children.* Austin, Tex:PRO-ED; 1987.

25. Weber B. Assessing low frequency hearing using auditory evoked potentials. *Ear Hear.* 1987;8(4):49S–54S.
26. Kileny P. Auditory brainstem responses as indicators of hearing aid performance. *Ann Otol Rhinol Laryngol.* 1982;238:233–240.
27. Beauchaine K, Gorga M. Applications of the auditory brainstem response to pediatric hearing aid selection. *Semin Hear.* 1988;9(1):61–73.
28. Matkin N. Wearable amplification: A litany of persisting problems. In Jerger J, ed. Pediatric Audiology. San Diego: College Hill Press; 1984.
29. Ross M. Binaural versus monaural hearing aids. In: Bess F, ed. *Childhood Deafness: Causation, Assessment, and Management.* New York: Grune & Stratton; 1977.
30. Matkin N. Hearing aids for children. In: Hodgson W, ed. *Hearing Aid Assessment and Use in Audiologic Habilitation.* Baltimore: Williams & Wilkins; 1986.
31. Luterman D. Counseling parents. In: Martin F, ed. *Hearing Disorders in Children.* Austin, Tex: PRO-ED; 1987.
32. Luterman D. *Counseling the Communicatively Disordered and Their Families.* Boston: Little, Brown; 1984.
33. Owens D, Kessler D. *Cochlear Implants in Young Deaf Children.* Boston: College-Hill; 1989.
34. Lynch M, Eilers R, Oller DK. Profoundly hearing impaired subjects: use of tactile aids in speech perception tasks. *Volta Rev.* 1989;91(5):113–126.
35. McGarr N, ed. Research on the use of sensory aids for hearing-impaired people. *Volta Rev.* 1989;91(5):1–138.
36. Simmons F. Diagnosis and rehabilitation of deaf newborns, Part II. *Asha.* 1980;22:475–479.
37. Ling D, Ling A. *Aural Habilitation: The Foundations of Verbal Learning in Hearing Impaired Children.* Washington, DC: A.G. Bell Association for the Deaf; 1978.
38. Luterman D. *Counseling Parents of Hearing Impaired Children.* Boston: Little, Brown; 1979.
39. Matkin N. Key considerations in counseling parents of hearing impaired children. *Semin Speech and Language.* 1988;9:209–222.
40. Robinson D, Sterling G. Hearing aids and children in school: a follow-up study. *Volta Rev.* 1980;82:229–235.
41. Hawkins D, Yacullo W. Signal-to-noise advantage of binaural hearing aids and directional microphones under different levels of reverberation. *J Speech Hear Disord.* 1984;49:278–286.
42. Bailey D. Issues and directions in preparing professionals to work with young handicapped children and their families. In: Gallagher J, Trohanis P, Clifford R, eds. *Policy Implementation and PL 99-457.* Baltimore: Paul H. Brookes; 1989.

Implementing the modified barium swallow evaluation in children who have multiple disabilities

Catherine A. Fox, MS, OTR/L
Coodinator
Feeding and Growth Management Program
Children's Hospital
Omaha, Nebraska

THE MODIFIED barium swallow is the radiographic procedure of choice for evaluating the swallowing mechanism. It differs from the standard barium swallow, which uses liquid barium to document the anatomy and physiology of the gastrointestinal system. During the modified barium swallow, a variety of factors are evaluated for their impact on the passage of food and liquids through the oral, pharyngeal, and cervical esophageal phases of the swallow. Indirect observation by videofluoroscopy during the procedure provides information on the quality of movement, degree of dysfunction, and degree of aspiration, as well as the effect of swallowing reeducation and compensatory techniques. Because of the closed nature of the swallowing mechanism, the modified barium swallow provides valuable information and thus assists in the development of effective feeding and swallowing programs. This article will review the swallowing process, the clinical indications for performing a modified barium swallow, and the specific evaluation techniques used with infants and children who have multiple disabilities.

NORMAL SWALLOWING

The swallowing process consists of highly synchronized sensory and motor events that move a bolus safely from the oral cavity to the stomach. This process is typically described in at least three phases: oral, pharyngeal, and esophageal. Although dysfunction in either the pharyngeal or esophageal phase of swallowing may be more life-threatening, clinical assessment has primarily focused on the oral phase because of its higher visibility.

Development of the swallowing mechanism involves the maturation of the central nervous system and the growth and elongation of the oral and pharyngeal structures. These structures in the newborn differ significantly from those in an adult; the former are characterized by a small oral space, large tongue, small recessed mandible, large buccal pads, large arytenoid cartilages, and high anterior position of the larynx[1] (Fig 1). These structures undergo rapid changes in size and

The author acknowledges Dr Wilbur Smith for his review of this article; Patricia Bahr for assistance in refining the positioning system prototype; Richard T. Huber for rendering the schematic of the prototype; and Nancy Knebel for secretarial support.

Inf Young Children 1990; 3(2): 67–77

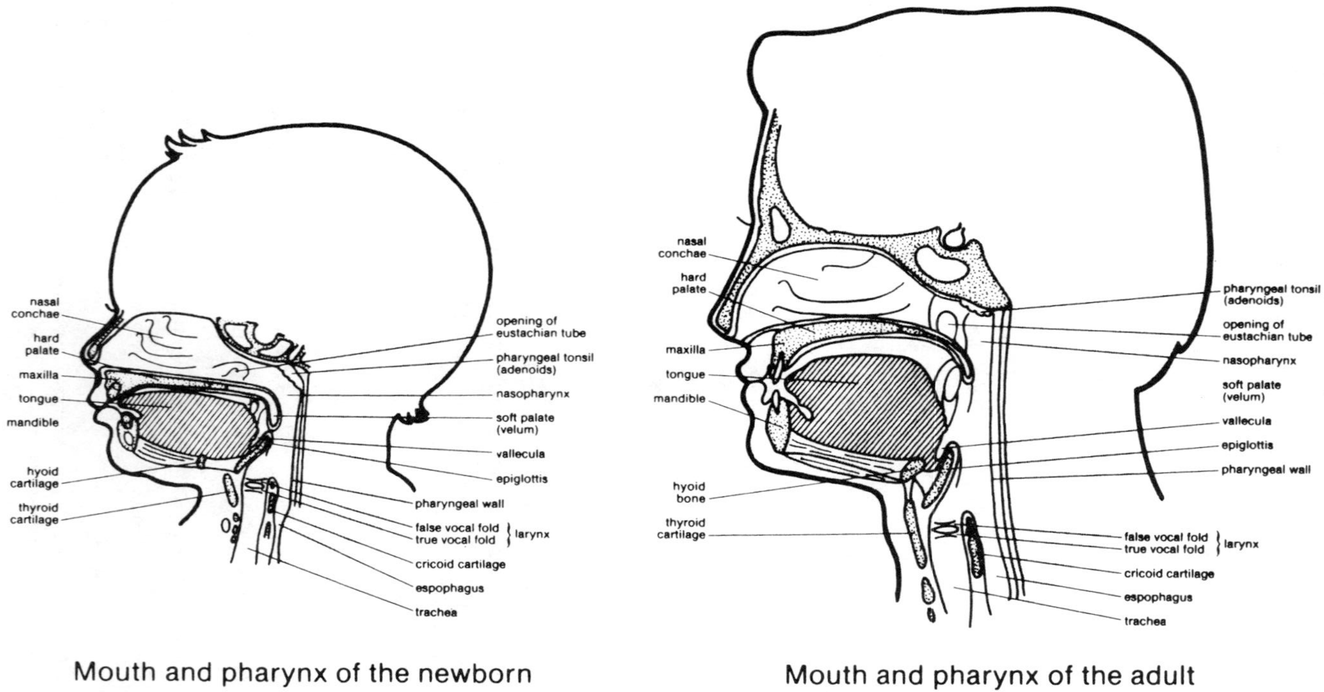

Fig 1. Anatomical differences between the newborn and the adult mouth and pharynx. *Source:* From *Pre-Feeding Skills* by Marsha Dunn Klein and Suzanne Evans Morris, copyright © 1987 by Therapy Skill Builders, a division of Communication Skill Builders, Inc., P.O. Box 42050, Tucson, AZ 85733. Reprinted with permission.

alignment during the first 4 years of life, and growth continues through puberty.[1] The number of phases in the swallowing process remains consistent from infancy through adulthood. The motor patterns within each phase, however, change as the child matures. The oral phase of infant swallow is characterized by the suckle pattern, which involves movement of the lower jaw and tongue against the palate and upper jaw. The tongue conforms around the nipple (of the breast or bottle) as the lips and mandible move down synchronously to create a negative intraoral pressure to express the fluid from the nipple. Swallowing of the liquid bolus is accomplished safely and efficiently by virtue of the mechanical alignment of the larynx under the base of the tongue and the large arytenoid cartilages.

Suckling evolves into transitional feeding patterns between 6 and 36 months of age and is characterized by isolated control of the tongue and jaw to manipulate higher food textures.[1] Feeding changes during this time from a stimulus-generated physiologic response to a self-directed activity that is shaped further by social and behavioral cues occurring around the feeding situation.

The mature oral phase has two components: the bolus preparation phase and the voluntary swallow phase. Bolus preparation includes adaptation of bolus consistency in terms of viscosity, elasticity, volume, mass, and temperature.[2] Food is manipulated and gathered into a bolus that is held between the tongue and anterior hard palate before voluntary initiation of the swallow. The pharyngeal airway is open during the oral preparatory phases, which makes it possible for a poorly managed bolus to enter the pharynx and possibly the trachea; this results in aspiration before the swallow.[3,4] Elevation of the tongue begins the voluntary swallow phase, during which the bolus is propelled posteriorly until it reaches the oropharynx. Once there, the bolus stimulates sensory receptors, which trigger the involuntary swallow reflex, thus ending the oral phase. The voluntary swallow phase takes less than 1 second to complete.

The pharyngeal phase begins when the swallow reflex is triggered. The soft palate elevates and retracts to close the nasopharynx, thus preventing food from entering the nasal cavity. The pharyngeal constrictor muscles work in coordination with all other structures to propel the bolus through the pharynx to the upper esophageal sphincter. This movement is peristaltic in nature and initiates the esophageal wave. Laryngeal closure occurs when the larynx is elevated and the epiglottis tips posteriorly closing the laryngeal vestibule and glottis, preventing the bolus from entering the trachea. During these events, there is a brief inhibition of respiration. The bolus then traverses the upper esophageal sphincter, which is relaxed for 1 second or less.

The esophageal phase begins with passage of the bolus through the upper esophageal sphincter into the esophagus. The bolus is carried by a distinct peristaltic wave through the esophagus to the gastroesophageal junction. This takes approximately 8 to 20 seconds.

DYSFUNCTIONAL SWALLOWING

Deviation in either the order or the quality of the physiologic movements during the oral and pharyngeal phases of the swallow may lead to dysfunctional swallowing and, possibly, to laryngeal penetration (ie, choking). Many factors have been identified as possible causes of swallowing disorders, including age, presence of disease, decreased consciousness, and abnormal anatomic structures. These factors alter the normal physiologic process through

- disturbances in motility,
- residual filling of recesses,
- stasis or pooling, and
- misdirected swallowing.[5]

Disturbances in motility may include partial or complete loss, delayed initiation, or prolonged duration of movements. Any one of these may alter the sequential order of the swallowing process and result in laryngeal penetration. Residual filling of the pharyngeal recesses may result from decreased sensation, motor deficiencies, or mechanical obstruction. Pooling in the vallecula, which cannot be seen clinically, is frequently evident on radiographic studies and is a distinct indicator of pharyngeal dysfunction. Pharyngeal stasis is the slowing or stopping of a bolus in structures within the pharynx, such as the pyriform sinuses. Aspiration, or what is referred to as misdirected swallowing, is the most striking abnormality observed clinically and radiographically[5] (Fig 2). Bolus deviation into the nasal cavity occurs when there is impaired closure of the nasopharynx.

The major cause of morbidity and mortality in adult patients with swallowing dysfunction is the aspiration of foreign material into the airway and lungs.[6] It should be noted that even normal individuals may have transient swallowing dysfunction that results in laryngeal penetration, but this dysfunction rarely causes problems, because of functional protective reflexes. This fact alone differentiates the functional from the dysfunctional swallower.

The evaluation and treatment of swallowing disorders is complex and increases in complexity with children. Consideration must be given to the

- anatomic and functional growth of the swallowing apparatus,
- maturation of the feeding behavior,
- oral feeding and the development of parent–child bonding,
- nutritional adequacy for growth, and
- limited cognitive ability (in certain high-risk groups).[7]

All of these factors have a significant impact on the child's ability to develop functional feeding and swallowing skills. Considerations for the child with multiple disabilities must also include the effects of delayed maturation of the central nervous system, abnormal neuromuscular control, and congenital or developing anatomical deformities.

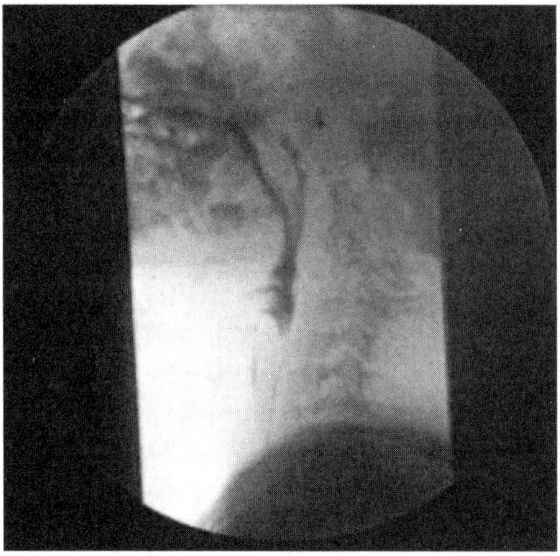

Fig 2. Radiograph showing nasopharyngeal reflux and airway penetration.

There are some children with multiple disabilities who have difficulty feeding from infancy, but who gain the necessary coordination to obtain and maintain a functional feeding status. Still other children with multiple disabilities, who initially have coordinated sucking and swallowing functions, eventually lose those functions as their neurologic maturation is unable to keep pace with the rapid structural growth and elongation in the oral and pharyngeal cavities. Swallowing disorders are frequently found in children with diffuse neurologic damage, whether congenital or acquired. The etiology of the problem may vary, but the sequela of dysfunctional swallowing remains. These children often experience repeated episodes of aspiration, recurrent pneumonia, and chronic lung disease, with corresponding poor oral intake and the possible development of protein energy malnutrition as well as subsequent immunologic compromise.[8] Feeding the child with multiple disabilities is often associated with long, laborious hours of using difficult feeding techniques; with slow oral intake, poor nutrition and hydration, coughing and choking, and behavior problems; and with the resulting frustration, anxiety, and guilt on the part of the caregivers.

DIAGNOSING SWALLOWING DYSFUNCTION

The diagnosis of swallowing dysfunction usually occurs in a four-step process including (1) a detailed review of the history, (2) a clinical evaluation, (3) a radiographic evaluation of the swallowing process, and (4) analysis of data. Adult patients have been able to describe with 99.2% accuracy symptoms that were consistent with the findings of radiographic studies.[4] Perhaps it is worth noting that such adults had experience with normal swallowing and then lost function, whereas children may have had limited or no experience with swallowing and have limited verbal abilities to describe symptoms. In the case of children, less direct information can be obtained about the nature of the swallowing problem, and more attention should be directed toward the child's history. Parents or caregivers may provide information about past and present feeding patterns, including preferred or best managed textures; medical history, including respiratory and gastrointestinal problems; cognitive level and ability to follow instructions; nutrition and hydration status; and the current medication regimen.

Clinical evaluation

The clinical examination of a child with multiple disabilities should provide information on

- general neuromotor status,
- postural deformities,
- oral structures,
- oral reflexes (ie, rooting, gag, suck/swallow),
- oral motor patterns of the tongue, lips, cheeks, and palate,
- oral sensations,
- laryngeal function (voice quality),
- current respiratory pattern,
- best food consistency for liquids and solids,
- best method of presenting liquids and solids,
- best feeding position,
- ability to follow directions and cooperate, and
- symptoms observed during the swallowing process.[9,10]

From the child's history, the swallowing therapist may be able to localize the phase or phases involved in the dysfunction, determine the easiest and most difficult textures to manage, and gain some indication of the pathophysiology of the swallowing disorder.[4,11] The clinical examination provides basic information for setting up and performing the modified barium swallow study. The swallowing therapist should identify

- the posture that may maximize swallowing abilities,
- the most effective method of presenting liquids and solids,
- the best textures of liquids and solids, and
- a sequence of presenting the textures to document the swallow function and maximize the information received during the study.[4,12]

Accurate prediction of laryngeal penetration is difficult because of the closed nature of the swallowing process. Studies[4,11] have shown that silent (undetected) aspiration was found in approximately 60% of adult patients who aspirated during radiographic studies.[4,11] A high incidence of silent aspiration has also been found during radiographic studies involving children with multiple disabilities.[13] All of these studies document the limitations of the clinical examination and emphasize the need for radiographic evaluation of the swallowing process.

Radiographic evaluation

The modified barium swallow has become an essential part of evaluating the swallow, determining swallowing reeducation techniques, and assessing treatment efficacy. Two primary imaging techniques include cineradiography and videofluoroscopy, each of which uses barium contrast for dynamic recording of the swallowing process. Cineradiography is recorded on motion picture film and provides sharper imaging via 60 frame-per-second analysis. Its limitations include increased radiation exposure, the time and cost of film development, and the difficulty of recording sound on the film. Videofluoroscopy is the imaging technique of choice for children, because of its lower radiation exposure. It is also less expensive and provides immediate playback, frame-by-frame or regular-speed analysis, ease of voice recording, and storage capabilities. Videoflouroscopy's imaging quality is slightly grainier, with only 30 frames-per-second analysis, but it provides adequate analysis capabilities.[4,14,15]

The modified barium swallow focuses on the structures involved in the swallowing process. This procedure dynamically records the anatomy and physiology of the oral, pharyngeal, and esophageal phases of the swallow during the ingestion of barium-impregnated food and drink. Each patient is evaluated for disturbances in motility, pooling in the pharyngeal recesses, and misdirection of the swallow. Accurate identification of compensation and decompensation patterns enables the delineation of effective treatment techniques.[5]

During the modified barium swallow evaluation, a variety of factors should be assessed to determine their impact on the swallowing mechanism. These factors include

- postural variations,
- head and neck position,
- bolus texture,
- bolus size,
- variations in the order of foods given,
- dry swallows (swallows without food or liquid),
- bolus placement in the mouth, and
- respiration patterns (ie, supraglottic swallow).

These factors can be used in any combination and can be implemented as compensation or reeducation techniques based on the anatomy and physiology that are present.[12,16]

Postural variations of the body, head, and neck affect the control and flow of food and liquid through the oral and pharyngeal cavities. Changes in head and neck positions alter the relationship of structures within the pharyngeal cavity to compensate for decreased motility; that is, as the child's body position in space changes, gravity becomes more of a factor. However, postural variations are considered to be compensatory techniques and do not necessarily improve the underlying physiologic function of the swallow.[8] Postural alignment can also influence the presence of primitive reflexes and abnormal muscle tone in children with multiple disabilities.

Bolus texture and size may be altered to facilitate improved oral and pharyngeal control. A larger bolus may help stimulate the swallow reflex; however, competent airway protection must be present, or penetration may occur. Using a smaller bolus in combination with neck flexion may prevent aspiration before the swallow by collecting the bolus in the vallecula until the swallow reflex is triggered. Bolus textures may be altered according to the properties that must be considered to determine the total impact on the swallow, based on the physiology in the oral and pharyngeal phases. Varying the placement of the bolus within the oral cavity can assist with decreased oral phase control, and alternating liquids and solids and using dry swallows may assist with the clearance of residue in the pharynx.[1,4,12] Specific respiration patterns such as the supraglottic swallow can be used to clear food particles from the larynx, although cognitive understanding of verbal commands is required.[12]

This evaluation can be obtained from either a lateral or antero/posterior viewpoint. From the lateral viewpoint, the movements of the lips, tongue, palate, epiglottis, and laryngeal structures; the contraction of pharyngeal musculature; and the opening of the upper esophageal sphincter can be observed. Oral and pharyngeal transit time, the mechanism of laryngeal penetration, and the degree of aspiration also are easily documented from this viewpoint. The antero/posterior viewpoint is used to document symmetry and bolus displacement and to obtain further assessment of the upper esophageal sphincter.[17]

The request for a swallowing evaluation may come from any person involved in the care of a child with multiple disabilities. The primary physician may evaluate the child or refer him or her to a team specializing in the evaluation and treatment of feeding and swallowing disorders. This team may include a variety of professionals, with the core team consisting of a physician, an occupational therapist and/or a speech pathologist, a behavior psychologist, a nutritionist, and a radiologist. The recommendation for a modified barium swallow is based on information obtained from the child's history and a thorough clinical evaluation. The presence of one or more of the following symptoms may establish the need for a modified barium swallow evaluation:

- frequent or recurrent pneumonia,
- infiltrates on a chest x-ray,
- recurrent upper respiratory infections not epidemic in nature,
- chronic lung changes,
- frequent or recurrent low-grade fevers,
- coughing while ingesting solids or liquids,
- increased congestion during and after feedings,
- change in voice quality during feedings (wet voice),
- decreased oral intake,
- poor weight gain or weight loss,
- food refusal,
- irritability during feedings,
- poor oral secretion control,
- sleepiness during or after meals,
- neuromotor involvement, and
- structural problems in the oral and/or pharyngeal mechanisms.

Unless the child has a dramatic clinical presentation, discrete symptoms of swallowing dysfunction may be overlooked. Therefore, detailed knowledge of clinical symptoms is important to enable the team to plan a radiographic evaluation that provides maximal diagnostic results while minimizing the amount of radiation exposure and potential for barium aspiration.

Orienting the child and family to the clinical and radiographic evaluation procedures is a necessary and effective way of reducing anxiety and obtaining trust and cooperation from the child and the family. Children often become anxious in the radiology suite but will tolerate the procedures fairly well if a reassuring, playful approach is used. Having the parent feed the child may further reduce the child's anxiety and incorporates the family into the evaluation procedures. Parental anxiety is generally directed toward the evaluation results, which may determine if the child should continue to be fed orally. These results are typically presented in an all-or-nothing manner on the basis of the presence or absence of airway penetration. A focus on what the child has or needs to gain in order to have a safe swallow allows the results to be communicated in a realistic yet positive manner. Family involvement facilitates better understanding of the child's immediate needs as well as the development of realistic treatment goals.

MODIFIED BARIUM SWALLOW PROCEDURES

Prior to the evaluation, these steps should be taken:

1. Meals may be withheld for at least 4 hours before the evaluation to increase the child's eagerness to eat and drink during the evaluation and to reduce the risk of vomiting and aspirating food during the study.
2. A chest film should be taken to document the status of the lungs. Chest films taken within 24 hours of the evaluation may be used if the child's clinical status

has not changed. It may be beneficial to have the child's caregiver involved in undressing and positioning the child, to minimize the child's anxiety.

3. The child's feeding utensils should be available for use during the evaluation.

4. The premature or very young infant may be positioned lying on the side within a warming nest on the x-ray table. The nest is created with three plastic sacks filled with warm water, which are placed on either side of the infant's trunk and at his or her feet. The area inside the nest is padded with a small blanket. This set-up gives small infants boundaries and reduces their environment, thus enabling them to quiet themselves. Their position within the nest can be changed and the effect of gravity on the swallowing mechanism can be evaluated by changing the angle of the x-ray table in space.

The young child's own positioning system should be evaluated for use with the imaging equipment. Visualization of the oral and pharyngeal structures must be unimpeded by head rests or other support systems. Several evaluation chairs have been designed to meet general imaging and positioning needs, but they are not suitable for patients with significant neuromotor involvement.[12] The child with multiple disabilities requires positioning equipment that can be individually fitted for the evaluation to provide maximum stability to the pelvis, trunk, and head, to assist with control of the child's muscle tone, and to maximize postural alignment, while providing comfort and security during the evaluation (Figs 3, 4). The positioning equipment should be placed as close as possible to the imaging equipment to reduce the amount of radiation scatter, to maximize the quality of the radiographic image, and to reduce the amount of image magnification (Fig 5).

5. A lead shield should be placed across the child's pelvis.

6. Numbers may be placed within the imaging field in the upper corner to identify changes in bolus texture and techniques.

7. The evaluation materials should include two syringes with 2 cc of thin liquid barium; two syringes with 2 cc of barium sulfate paste; the child's bottle or cup containing thin barium; two of the child's spoons prepared with 2 cc of barium sulfate paste, in semisolid form (rice cereal mixed with thin liquid barium); and a cookie covered with barium sulfate paste. The evaluation textures are based on the child's current diet and results of the clinical evaluation.

During the evaluation these steps are taken:

1. The premature or small infant should be positioned lying on the side, and the young child should be positioned as upright as possible for a lateral view.

2. The person feeding the child should be familiar with his or her feeding patterns and the current feeding techniques.

3. The modified barium swallow evaluation follows currently established guidelines.[4,12,15,16] The initial goal of the evaluation is to document the quality of the airway protection and the mechanism of dysfunction. In the lateral view, the imaging field should exclude the orbits and focus initially on the oral and pharyn-

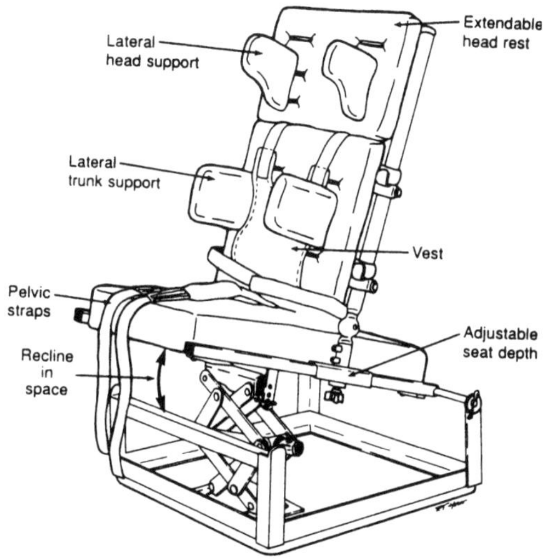

Fig 3. Schematic drawing of a positioning system prototype, designed for use during the modified barium swallow in children who have multiple disabilities. Reprinted with permission. © 1990 Catherine A. Fox.

geal cavities, including the soft palate, and then the pharynx and the cervical esophagus.[16] Once the quality of airway protection is documented, the imaging field may be changed to document other components of the swallowing process, such as the oral phase. Esophageal motility should be evaluated only after the oral and pharyngeal phases have been well documented.

4. The small infant should be given a bottle of thin barium, adapted with the nipple of choice, and allowed to suckle. Alternation of bottle and pacifier allows documentation of the nonnutritive suckle along with clearing of the oral and pharyngeal cavities. Evaluation of the small child should begin with administration of 2 cc of liquid barium to allow documentation of the quality of the swallowing mechanism. If appropriate, a second liquid bolus may be given or the evaluation may proceed to the texture that is best-managed clinically.

5. Compensation and swallowing reeducation techniques should be evaluated on the basis of decompensation patterns noted during the initial swallow of each texture.

6. Once the swallowing process has been documented, the child should be fed in the manner and position of a typical meal, unless significant aspiration has been previously noted. The antero/posterior viewpoint may be attempted if specific asymmetries are suspected, but this position is difficult for a child with multiple disabilities, becuase of poor head and neck control.

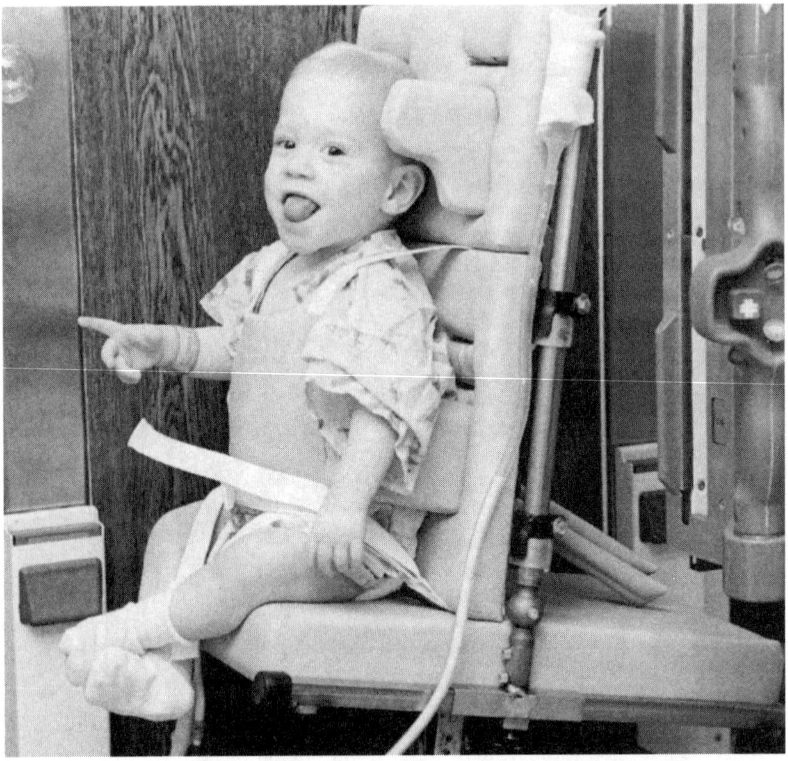

Fig 4. Positioning system prototype set up on foot board of x-ray table.

After the evaluation these steps should be taken:

1. A chest film should be taken to determine the status of the lungs and the extent of aspiration. If significant aspiration has occurred, postural drainage and chest percussion may be used to help clear the lung.
2. The radiologist and members of the feeding team should analyze the evaluation tape, in order to make treatment decisions and recommendations.
3. The parents and caregivers are instructed to give plenty of fluids and a laxative to assist with passage of the barium through the gastrointestinal tract.

TREATMENT AND FOLLOW-UP

For many children with multiple disabilities, reeducation of their swallowing mechanism will be a slow developmental process because of the nature of their

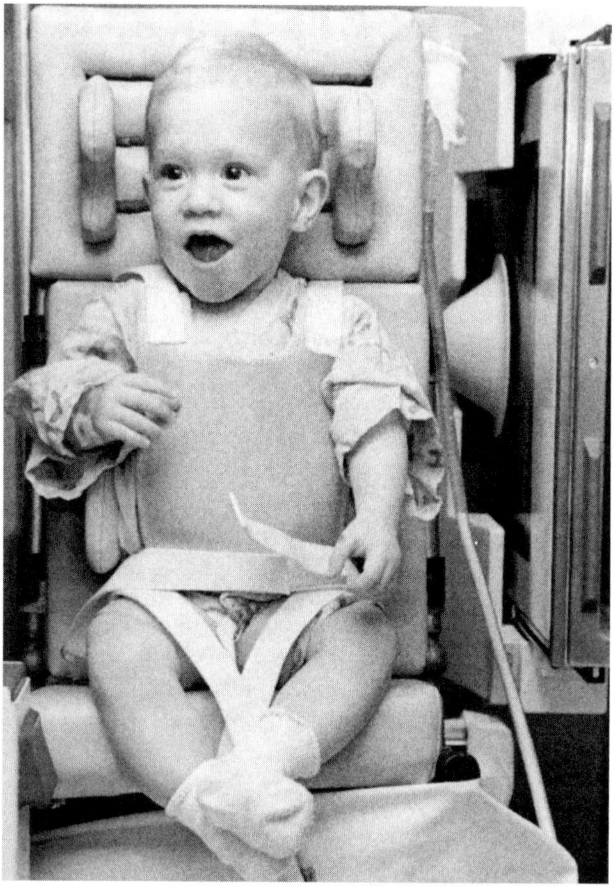

Fig 5. The relationship of the positioning system to the x-ray table enhances the quality of the radiographic evaluation and reduces radiation scatter.

brain damage. By using the modified barium swallow with slow-motion analysis, the feeding team should be able to delineate the area and degree of dysfunction, as well as the effect of swallowing compensations and reeducation techniques. The recommended techniques should be reviewed for their impact on the length of time required to feed a meal, the child's energy expenditure, and the child's ability to meet daily nutrition and hydration requirements. To establish a realistic feeding program, consideration must also be given to the child's behavioral characteristics and the caregivers' capabilities in terms of skill and time.

It is not uncommon for children with multiple disabilities to be able to manage only a limited range of food textures. As a result, manipulation of the nutritional content of the child's diet or supplementation with partial or total tube feeding represent management options that may be used to establish a feeding program that is safe, nutritionally appropriate, and realistic, while maintaining some oral and pharyngeal stimulation activities.

Reevaluation of the child's swallowing mechanism should be a periodic part of treatment management and follow-up. Repeat evaluations should be considered if there is a significant change in the child's medical or neurologic status, if previous symptoms recur, if silent aspiration was previously documented, and if a significant change in the feeding program involving compensation techniques or diet textures is indicated. The frequency of the reevaluation should be based on the speed and degree of clinical change.

• • •

The closed nature and complexity of the swallowing mechanism can be safely evaluated with the modified barium swallow under videofluoroscopy. This evaluation identifies penetration and aspiration and provides detailed information about the degree of dysfunction. More important, it documents the quality of the swallow and the impact on the swallowing mechanism of compensations and reeducation techniques. The feeding team is then able to prescribe a nutritionally complete feeding program that maximizes the child's oral capabilities, while placing realistic demands on the caregivers and the child with multiple disabilities.

REFERENCES

1. Bosma J. Development of feeding. *Clin Nutr.* 1986;5:210–218.
2. Buchhols D, Bosma J, Donner M. Adaptations, compensation, and decompensation of the pharyngeal swallow. *Gastrointes Radiol.* 1985;10:235–239.
3. Curtis D, Hudson T. Laryngotracheal aspiration: Analysis of specific neuromuscular factors. *Radiology.* 1983;149:517–522.
4. Logemann J. *Evaluation and Treatment of Swallowing Disorders.* San Diego: College-Hill Press, Inc., 1983.
5. Donner M, Silbiger M. Cinefluorographic analysis of pharyngeal swallowing in neuromuscular disorders. *Am J Med Sci.* 1966;140:600–615.
6. Zimmerman J, Oder L. Swallowing dysfunction in acutely ill patients. *Phys Ther.* 1981;61:1755–1763.
7. Tuchman D. Dysfunctional swallowing in the pediatric patient: Clinical considerations. *Dysphagia.* 1988;2:203–208.
8. MacLean WC. Protein-energy malnutrition (PEM). In: MacLean WC, Graham G, eds. *Pediatric Nutrition in Clinical Practice.* Menlo Park, Calif: Addison-Wesley, 1982.

9. Griggs C, Jones P, Lee R. Videofluoroscopic investigations of feeding disorders of children with multiple handicaps. *Dev Med Child Neurol.* 1989;31:303–307.
10. Kenny D, Koheil R, Greenberg J, et al. Development of a multidisciplinary feeding profile for children who are dependent feeders. *Dysphagia.* 1989;4:16–28.
11. Splaingard M, Hutchins B, Sulton L, Chaudhuri B. Aspiration in rehabilitation patients: Videofluoroscopy vs. bedside clinical assessment. *Arch Phys Med Rehabil.* 1988;60:637–640.
12. Logemann J. *Manual for the Videofluorographic Study of Swallowing.* San Diego: College-Hill Press, Inc., 1986.
13. Helfrich-Miller K, Rector K, Straka J. Dysphagia: Its treatment in the profoundly retarded patient with cerebral palsy. *Arch Phys Med Rehabil.* 1986;31:303–307.
14. Donner M, Jones B. Gastrointestinal radiology. *Gastrointest Radiol.* 1985;10:195–211.
15. Sorin R, Somers S, Austin W, Bester S. The influence of videofluoroscopy on the management of the dysphagic patient. *Dysphagia.* 1988;2:127–135.
16. Siebens A, Linden P. Dynamic imaging for swallowing re-education. *Gastrointest Radiol.* 1985;10:251–253.
17. Jones B, Kramer S, Donner M. Dynamic imaging of the pharynx. *Gastrointest Radiol.* 1985;10:213–224.

Safe transportation for infants and preschoolers with special needs

Janet D. Stout, MS, OTR
Assistant Professor of Occupational Therapy
Indiana University School of Medicine
Indianapolis, Indiana

Marilyn J. Bull, MD
Professor of Pediatrics
Indiana University School of Medicine
Director
Automotive Safety for Children Program
James Whitcomb Riley Hospital for Children
Indianapolis, Indiana

Karen Bruner Stroup, PhD
Research Associate
Automotive Safety for Children Program
James Whitcomb Riley Hospital for Children
Indianapolis, Indiana

WITHIN THE last decade the safe transportation of young children has improved due to a combination of legislation, increased public awareness, and improved products. In addition, there is more literature available to guide interdisciplinary teams of health care providers in developing and providing safe restraint for children with special needs.[1] The child safety seat or "car seat" has come to be accepted as a standard piece of equipment for infants, toddlers, and preschool-age children. Despite the increased use of car seats,[2] however, motor vehicle accidents remain a leading cause of death and injury among young children.[3] Several studies suggest that the misuse of restraints contributes significantly to the incidence of vehicle-related mortality and morbidity.[4–6]

There is a significant need for continued public education to reduce misuse of restraint systems, particularly with respect to the safe and proper restraint of children with special needs that prevent conventional use of standard car seats. These children unlike their nonhandicapped counterparts, remain at high risk of injury or death due not only to misuse but also to limited information, procedural guidelines, and suitably designed products. As a result, the use of makeshift restraints or no restraints is all too common. Children with orthopedic, neurologic, respiratory, or other medical problems often require special positioning and fitting considerations for proper restraint, causing parents and health care providers to modify standard restraints or to forego use of a child safety seat. Such actions significantly jeopardize the safety of these already medically fragile children during transportation.

The purpose of this article is (1) to review recent trends that have served as catalysts to development of safer means of transport for infants and young chil-

The authors express sincere appreciation to M & K Photography for photographs, to David G. Marrero, PhD, for editorial assistance, and to the Indiana Division of Traffic Safety for their support.

Inf Young Children 1989; 2(2): 67–73

dren; (2) to address medical concerns that interfere with safe transportation for special-needs children; and (3) to suggest guidelines for correcting these problems.

TRENDS TOWARD SAFER TRANSPORT OF INFANTS AND YOUNG CHILDREN

There is increasing national acknowledgment that the lives of our children should not be jeopardized by inadequate protection during transportation. By 1984 all states had passed legislation requiring the use of car restraints for young children. As a result of these laws, many states have reported decreases in fatalities and injuries to young children.[7,8]

In 1981, after massive research efforts, Federal Motor Vehicle Safety Standard (FMVSS) 213 (49 CFR 571.213 § 30,849E) was established to improve design and performance of car seats. FMVSS 213 specifies requirements for child restraint systems, such as shell thickness, padding density, head and knee excursion limits, separate securement for child and seat, and dynamic crash tolerances. FMVSS 213 applies to children weighing up to 50 lb. However, it does not specify a minimum occupant weight in its evaluation of the design and performance of car seats, nor does it address the needs of the developmentally delayed child over 50 lb. These concerns will be addressed later in this article.

In 1979 FMVSS 222 was developed to improve the safety of able-bodied children riding on school buses. FMVSS 222 established guidelines related to compartmentalization, seat height, and padding. Although FMVSS 222 does not address the needs of children who cannot ride safely on the conventional school bus, many states are responding on an individual basis to establish minimum specifications for special education school buses. Research by Schneider[9,10] and others[11,12] has provided an important basis for establishing minimum requirements, such as the forward-facing installation of wheelchairs.

Other legislation that has increased attention to safer transportation for children with special needs includes Public Laws 98-199 and 99-457, which amended the Education for All Handicapped Children Act of 1975 (Public Law 94-142). Public Law 98-199 of 1983 (the Education of the Handicapped Act Amendments) and Public Law 99-457 of 1986 (Handicapped Infants and Toddlers Amendments) provide financial assistance to enable states to begin providing educational opportunities for children from birth to 6 years of age. If school transportation is included in the implementation of these early intervention programs, the number of special-needs children requiring transportation restraints will increase dramatically. In order for these laws to meet their objectives fully, attention must be directed to the provision of safe transportation using restraints that are scientifically designed and evaluated.

RESEARCH ON RESTRAINTS FOR SPECIAL-NEEDS CHILDREN

Studies on safe transportation for special-needs children were virtually nonexistent until the mid 1980s. Since that time, however, several articles have addressed concerns related to special-needs infants and toddlers. Bull and Stroup[13] evaluated the dimensions of various child safety seats for premature infants and illustrated methods for increasing a premature infant's comfort and safety while in the car seat by adding rolled towels and cloth diapers for head and trunk support and to help prevent slouching. They found seats with shields to be unacceptable for premature infants.

Willett et al[14] evaluated 30 infants for ventilatory compromise in car seats and concluded that there may be risk of hypoxia for some premature infants. Since it is recognized that lap-held infants are at the greatest risk of injury, Willett et al recommended that low birth weight infants be monitored for transcutaneous or pulse oximetry in the chosen car seat before discharge from the nursery. It was further recommended that new car seat designs be developed for low birth weight infants to allow for prone or supine positioning.

Bull et al[15] recognized that there is no minimum child weight specification in FMVSS 213. An anthropomorphic dummy simulating a 6-month-old child weighing 17 lb (7.7 kg) is currently required for dynamic crash testing by FMVSS 213 to evaluate the performance restraint systems. The test dummy used in the Bull et al study was designed to simulate a 4.75-lb (2.1-kg) infant and was tested with four conventional semiupright rear-facing car seats, all of which effectively restrained the test dummy. These authors further evaluated the Swinger Car Bed (Fig 1) through dynamic crash testing to determine its suitability as a restraint system for premature infants whose medical condition requires that they be transported in a prone or supine position. A smaller bunting designed to restrain the infant weighing less than 5 lb inside the Swinger Car Bed was also designed, and it performed satisfactorily in crash testing.

The Swinger Car Bed has been recommended for infants with other medical conditions that necessitate prone or supine travel.[16] The Swinger accommodates infants weighing up to 20 lb (9.1 kg) and measuring less than 26 in long. Conditions necessitating this special positioning might include severe hydrocephalus, Pierre Robin syndrome, osteogenesis imperfecta, and body casting.

Safety seat use of children with hip spica casts has been addressed in the literature.[1,16–18] Treatment for congenitally dislocated hips (CDH) may include 3 to 12 months in a spica cast or brace, which holds the femurs in wide abduction and thus makes use of a conventional safety seat difficult if not impossible. Century child restraint models 100 and 300 (no longer commercially available) were modified for use with children with CDH, dynamically crash tested, and found to be uncompromised in performance as a restraint system.[17] The Modified Strolee 612 (Fig 2),

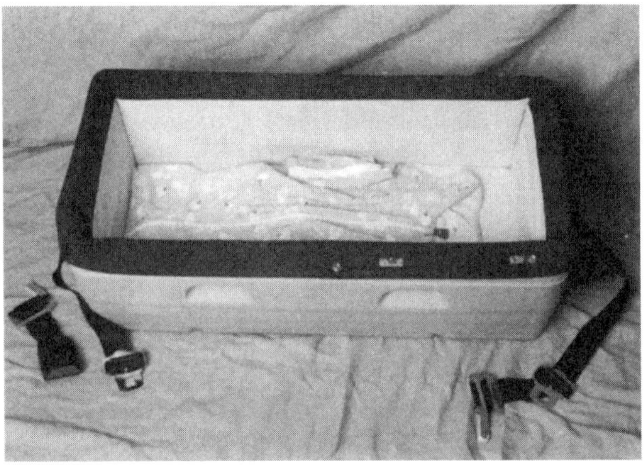

Fig 1. Swinger Car Bed.

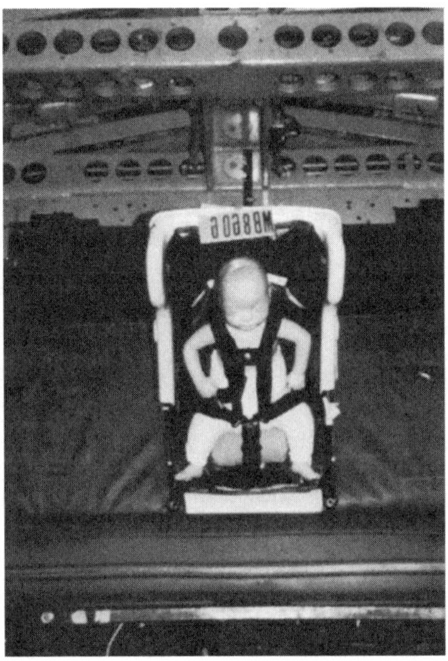

Fig 2. Modified Strolee 612.

Spelcast Car Seat (Fig 3), and Modified E-Z-On Vest M101 (Fig 4) were described as other suitable alternatives for various ages and sizes of children with CDH.[16]

Developmentally delayed children who weigh more than 40 lb are technically too large for most toddler car seats. If they lack head and trunk control they are not ready for booster seats, but there are several other commercially available options designed specifically for special-needs children.[16] Options include the Special Seat (Fig 5), the Orthopedic Positioning Seat, the Safety Rehab 500 (Fig 6) and 900 series Travel Chairs, the Ortho-Kinetics Travel Chair (Fig 7), the Carrie Car Seat (Fig 8), the Snug Seat (Fig 9), and the Kidster wheelchair (Fig 10).

The E-Z-On Vest is a multipurpose restraint that could be used for children with behavior problems, poor trunk control, or medical conditions necessitating prone or supine travel.[16] The vest can be modified by the manufacturer to include a crotch strap, posterior fastenings, or side loops for the prone/supine traveler.

As more children are being discharged from the hospital on ventilators, several special transportation concerns arise.[19] A seat with a shield could cause damage to the tracheostomy on impact. Regular car seats with five-point internal harness systems are appropriate for these children. A second concern is that of securing the oxygen and ventilator equipment during travel. Securement is recommended so that this equipment does not move precariously during sudden stops or a crash. Unsecured equipment could potentially injure other passengers as well as the ventilator-dependent child. To date there is no commercially available product for restraining ancillary medical equipment. Transportation specialists and health care providers must

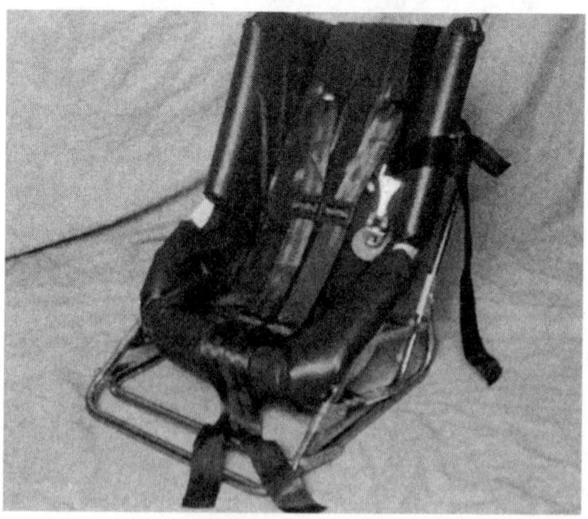

Fig 3. Spelcast Car Seat.

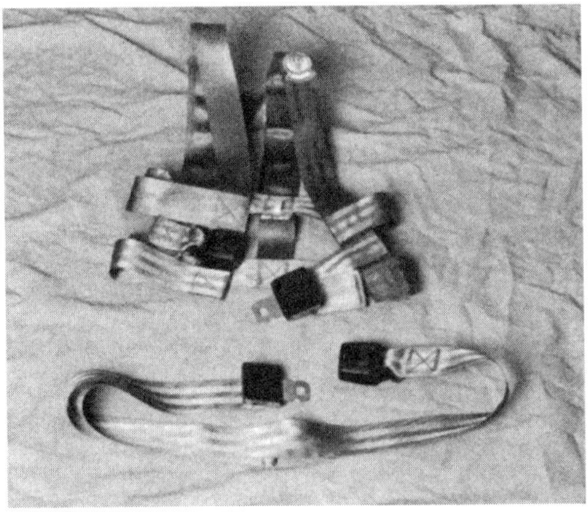

Fig 4. Modified E-Z-On Vest M101.

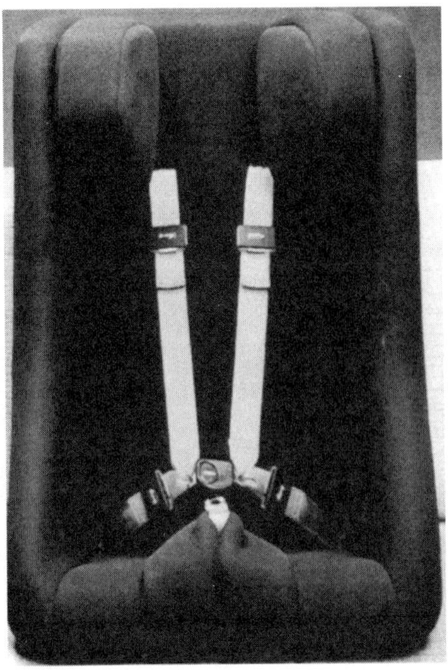

Fig 5. Special Seat.

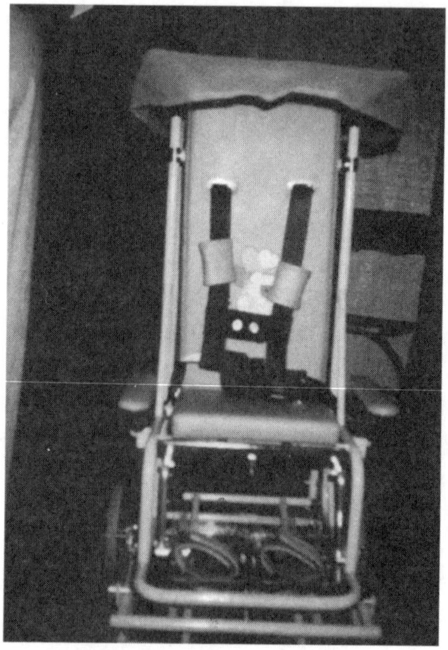

Fig 6. Safety Rehab 500 series Travel Chair.

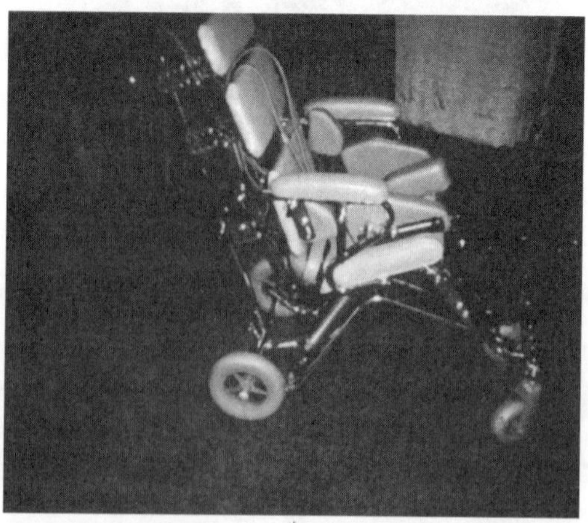

Fig 7. Ortho-Kinetics Travel Chair.

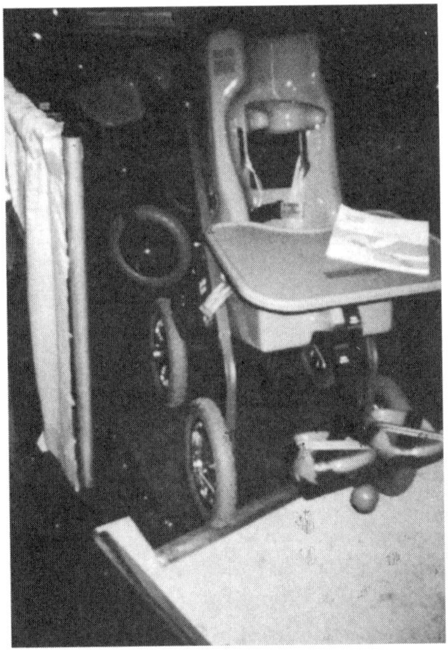

Fig 8. Carrie Car Seat.

therefore improvise solutions, which often entail the use of materials that have not been dynamically tested and may not be crashworthy. Equipment should not be positioned on a vehicle seat but on the floor, on the base of a wheelchair, secured to a school bus seat leg, or on the wall below window level. Until dynamically tested products become available, health care providers should rely on materials designed for securing products during transport, such as standard seat belts.

Wheelchair travel is of great concern to all those involved in the safe transportation of children,[9,12] but since it typically involves the older child, it is beyond the scope of this article. However, some general guidelines that may affect younger children are that (1) children weighing less than 30 lb should be secured in car seats, and (2) all children who can reasonably be transferred should be seated upright on a vehicle seat and secured with seat belts, with their wheelchairs secured separately.

• • •

Provision for the safe transportation of children with special needs is not yet comparable to the effort mounted to create acceptance of car seat and seat belt use

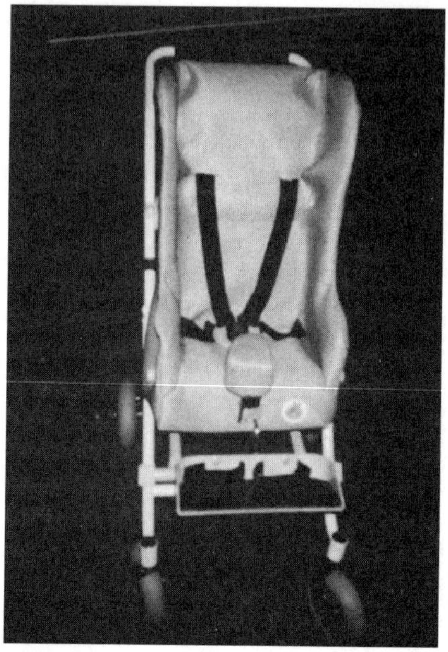

Fig 9. Snug Seat.

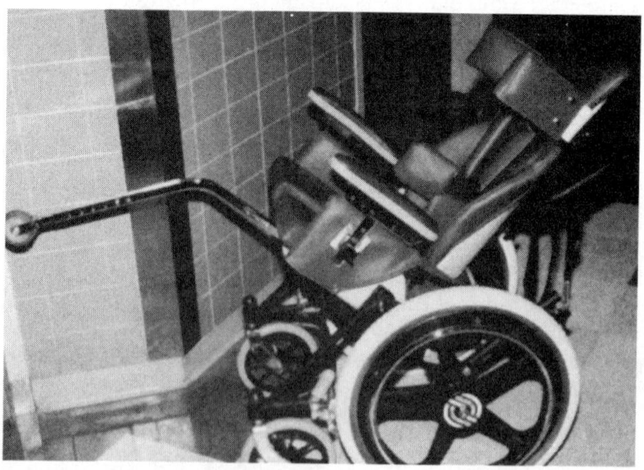

Fig 10. Kidster wheelchair.

for children without medical problems. All children are entitled to safe transportation and should not be secured in restraint systems that are substandard, makeshift, and incapable of withstanding crash forces. Parents and health care providers should not sanction the use of improvised restraints or of no restraints and should keep apprised of current research and dynamically tested transportation resources.

An interdisciplinary approach to providing safe transportation for children with special needs is vital. Families, physicians, nurses, occupational therapists, physical therapists, respiratory therapists, and transporters must work together to identify and achieve effective improvements in transportation safety.

REFERENCES

1. Feller N, Bull MJ, Gunnip A, et al: A multidisciplinary approach to developing safe transportation for children with special needs. *Orthop Nurs* 1986;5(5):25–27.
2. Restraint system usage in the traffic population, US Department of Transportation report No. DOT HS 807 342. Washington, DC, National Highway Traffic Safety Administration, 1988.
3. *Accident Facts.* Chicago, National Safety Council, 1988.
4. Cynecki MJ, Gocyl ME: The incidence and factors associated with child safety seat misuse, US Department of Transportation report No. DOT HS 806 676. Washington, DC, National Highway Traffic Safety Administration, 1984.
5. Agran PF: The effects of safety seat legislation on pediatric trauma, US Department of Transportation, Office of University Research report No. DTRS 5683–C–00027. Irvine, Calif, Public Policy Research Organization, 1985.
6. Bull MJ, Stroup KB, Gerhart S: Misuse of car safety seats. *Pediatrics* 1988;81:98–101.
7. Agran PF, Dunkle DE, Winn DG: Effects of legislation on motor vehicle injuries to children. *Am J Dis Child* 1987;141:959–962.
8. Margolis LH, Wagenaar AC, Liu W: The effects of a mandatory child restraint law on injuries requiring hospitalization. *Am J Dis Child* 1988;142:1099–1103.
9. Schneider LW: Protection for the severely disabled: A new challenge in occupant restraint, in *Proceedings of the International Symposium on Occupant Restraint.* Morton Grove, Ill, American Association for Automotive Medicine, 1981, pp 217–231.
10. Benson J, Schneider L: University of Michigan Transportation Research Institute: Improving the crashworthiness of restraints for handicapped children, Society of Automotive Engineers technical paper No. 840528. Warrendale, Pa, Society of Automotive Engineers, 1984.
11. Standards Association of Australia: Wheelchair occupant restraint assemblies for motor vehicles, Australian Standard 2942, Standards House, 80 Arthur Street, North Sydney, 1987.
12. Shaw G: Vehicular transport safety for the child with disabilities. *Am J Occup Ther* 1987;41:35–42.
13. Bull MJ, Stroup KB: Premature infants and car seats. *Pediatrics* 1985;75:336–339.
14. Willett LD, Leuschen MP, Nelson LS, et al: Risk of hypoventilation in premature infants in car seats. *J Pediatr* 1986;109:245–248.
15. Bull MJ, Weber K, Stroup KB: Automotive restraint systems for premature infants. *J Pediatr* 1988;112:385–388.

16. Stout JD, Bull MJ, Stroup KB: Safe transportation for children with disabilities. *Am J Occup Ther* 1989;43:31–36.

17. Bull MJ, Weber, K, Stroup KB: Safety seat use for children with hip dislocation. *Pediatrics* 1986;77:873–875.

18. Shesser LK: Car seat modification for children under treatment for congenital dislocated hips. *Orthop Nurs* 1985;4(6):11–13.

19. Stroup KB, Wylie P, Bull MJ: Car seats for children with mechanically assisted ventilation. *Pediatrics* 1987;80:290–292.

Information and referral for people with special needs: Implications for the Central Directory of Public Law 99-457

Kathy L. Mayfield-Smith, MA, MBA
Project Director

Girish G. Yajnik, MBA
Associate Director
Division of Information Technology

Denise L. Wiles, MSW
Project Director
Center for Developmental Disabilities
Department of Pediatrics
School of Medicine
University of South Carolina
Columbia, South Carolina

FAMILIES WITH children who have disabilities or delays in development face the usual issues of raising children, but they must also deal with a complex array of factors related to the children's special needs. These include such things as handling the excessive financial burden of frequent or extended medical care, finding special equipment, learning about a special condition or disability and what their child's special needs are, and learning which services are available to meet those needs. Their ability to meet these demands depends on their ability to access information about each of these diverse needs. Consequently, they have a much greater need for information and services than families of children without handicaps.[1]

Information and referral (I&R) is the method of connecting a person in need of a service or information source to the needed service or source. The multitude of services available and the complex requirements of these services create a situation in which it is not feasible for an individual or service provider to be aware of all specialized community services. Consequently, information and referral in today's society requires a professionally operated service dedicated to providing information.

Public Law 99-457—Education of the Handicapped Act, Amendments 1986[2]—mandates a central resource of information about services for families of infants and toddlers with developmental delays or disabilities. Part H of the law requires the statewide system to have "a central directory which includes early intervention services, resources, and experts available in the State, and research and demonstration projects being conducted in the State."[2(p1146)]

In considering the intent of this legislation, Silverstein states that "there is nothing more central than the family."[3(pA4)] Implementation of this law should emphasize that professionals work with individual families and respond to the unique

The operation of the SCSIS (South Carolina Services Information System) is supported by the State of South Carolina, the South Carolina Developmental Disabilities Council, the Department of Health and Environmental Control, and The University of South Carolina. The opinions expressed are those of the authors and do not necessarily represent those of the sponsors.

needs of each family. Two underlying concepts allow families to meet their own needs and meet the needs of their young child[4-6]: (1) *enabling,* which means creating opportunities for family members to develop skills necessary to meet their needs, and (2) *empowering,* which means assisting family members to develop a sense of control in the course of their lives. Information is a major tool that empowers families to act for themselves and to provide the highest quality of life possible for their family members with special needs.[7,8] In meeting the intent of Public Law 99-457, information should be provided to each family in a way that fits that individual family's needs. Some families may require only minimal information or the answer to a single question. Some may require small pieces of information over an extended period of time in order to access complex services. Other families may need different kinds of information to assist them through each transition period they face.

This article provides a brief background on information and referral and describes a model information and referral system for people with special needs and the system's applications under Public Law 99-457, Part H. In addition, a brief discussion of the issues related to implementing the central directory requirement is explored.

HISTORICAL PERSPECTIVE

Organized I&R services began in the early 1920s when social service exchanges[9-11] were established primarily to serve professionals. Not until the 1960s and 1970s did I&Rs begin to focus on the needs of consumers.[11] Since then, generic I&R services have proliferated; most serve local communities and focus on general human services. A few states (eg, Louisiana, Massachusetts, New Jersey, New Mexico, Oklahoma, and South Carolina) have centralized information about services for persons with disabilities and are easily accessible to families, especially those with low incomes.

The two primary functions of any I&R system continue to be (1) linking people in need with available and appropriate resources or services; and (2) assisting in long-range, systematic planning by using the data contained in the system to identify gaps and duplications in services.[9,10] The process of linking people with services varies from simply identifying the service provider and referring the inquirer, to providing ongoing information that helps the inquirer negotiate the maze of services, to advocating for the client who cannot get the needed services.[11]

For a person who wants to access available community services, the first step is to locate the desired services. The initial approach to this process was to print directories that could be used to find the needed service. Directories were supplemented by card files and brochures containing the services and providers that had been omitted from the directories. Inquiries were answered by leafing through the materials and searching out the replies to questions. A major problem for these manual systems was that their information was often out-of-date and incomplete because the printed materials required a long time to prepare and were too expensive to reproduce and distribute on a regular basis. Consequently, these materials were infrequently updated. An additional problem for manual I&R systems was the dramatic increase in the volume of information available and the concurrent increase in requests and in the time and the number of staff members required to respond to the requests.

Advancements in computer technology have provided solutions to some of the earlier I&R problems. Ten years ago systems were limited by the high costs of the equipment and the specialists needed to operate the equipment and the costs associated with developing the necessary software programs. This situation has improved. Lower hardware prices and the development of user-friendly software for microcomputer-driven databases have enabled some communities to provide I&R systems for their residents. Many of these systems are successful.

The professional literature supports the concept that I&R services are needed. People who need services may not get them, even when there is no charge for the service. Harris and Associates reported that "no more than 13 percent of the persons with disabilities have used these services, which are generally available throughout the country."[12(p18)] Bailey and Simeonsson[13] corroborate Harris's findings and state that there is an urgent need to inform persons about key services that are available to them. They state, "The greatest obstacle to information dissemination is the lack of a central resource center that can direct those in need of services to those who can provide the services."[13(p131)]

Public Law 99-457 mandated the provision of a central directory of information about services to meet the needs of families having very young children who either have or are at risk for developmental delays. The central directory provides the mechanism to enable families to have access to the information they need. For this mechanism to be effective, professionals and planners must work with each other and with families to ensure that the information that is needed by families is included and that the mechanism is accessible.[2]

A STATEWIDE MODEL FOR AN I&R SYSTEM

In South Carolina, the Center for Developmental Disabilities (CDD) has provided a central resource for information about services for persons with disabilities since 1982. The South Carolina Services Information System (SCSIS) is a computer-based information and referral system that provides information in response to requests received over a toll-free telephone line. This system was developed in response to a need identified by the South Carolina Developmental Disabilities Council to assist persons with developmental disabilities.

SCSIS is operated and administered by the CDD, Department of Pediatrics of the University of South Carolina School of Medicine. The CDD is part of the

University-Affiliated Program of South Carolina. Funding for the SCSIS combines resources from the State of South Carolina, the South Carolina Developmental Disabilities Council, the University of South Carolina, and private contributions.

Persons with special needs have complex and unique information requirements[1] that cannot be met by an I&R service designed for the general public. Therefore the primary focus of SCSIS has always been the consumer with special needs. While SCSIS does serve the needs of professionals, it was created for, and has continually evolved to respond to, the needs of parents, families, and individuals with disabilities.

The basic process of providing information and referral using this model is depicted in Fig 1. At the SCSIS, the information specialist begins by assessing the situation with the caller. The information specialist asks pertinent questions related to the caller's needs and documents relevant information (eg, client's age, gender, area or residence, disability, services requested). Once service needs are identified, the information specialist uses the computer to search for possible providers. By discussing each of the options with the caller, the information specialist provides referrals that meet the individual caller's needs. Often during the course of the call the needs for multiple services is identified. For example, the caller may request information about speech or physical therapy. Once the provider is identified, the information specialist may determine that the caller also needs transportation to get to the service and financial assistance to pay for the service. The information specialist repeats the process of searching for providers until all the information needs are met. If the services do not exist, these gaps are documented and included in reports to planners in the state.

The SCSIS database contains information about more than 5,500 providers of over 60,000 services in South Carolina. Three information specialists respond monthly to over 400 calls, resulting in approximately 775 referrals.

As the central information resource for persons with disabilities in South Carolina, SCSIS provides the framework for coordinating information about services. Its flexible design enables SCSIS to expand and incorporate specific information segments to address the needs of many specific groups with special needs. Service categories, handicapping conditions, and service providers unique to each special group can be added to the system as needed. As such, the SC Department of Health and Environmental Control, the lead agency for ensuring compliance with Public Law 99-457, Part H, has contracted with the Center for Developmental Disabilities to expand SCSIS to be the central directory.

COMPONENTS OF AN I&R SYSTEM

Formal standards for generic I&R services were developed by the United Way of America in 1973 and revised by the Alliance on Information and Referral Services in 1978 and again in 1983.[10] Although these standards provide an excellent

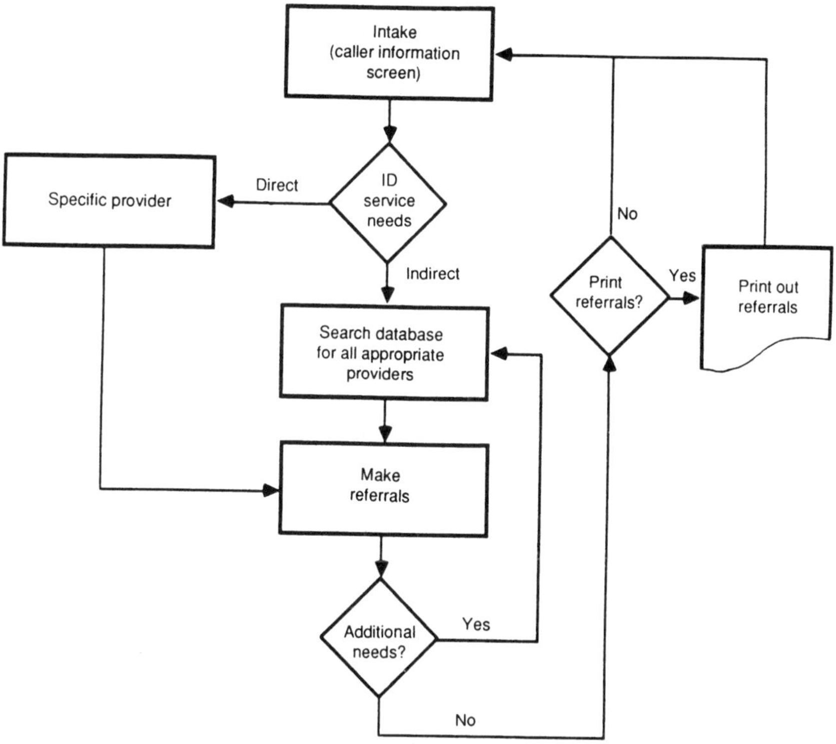

Fig 1. Flowchart of the referral process.

foundation, they do not sufficiently address the I&R needs of people with special needs, nor do they discuss computerized I&R systems. Many activities are involved in operating a successful I&R system. This article, however, will discuss only five major components that have enabled the South Carolina model to respond successfully to the needs of South Carolina citizens with disabilities:

- Database of information and resources
- Classification systems
- Accessibility to the I&R system
- Trained information specialists
- Computer

Database of information and resources

The information collected about organizations, services, and other resources is the foundation of the I&R system.[14] This information should be complete, accurate, up-to-date, and most of all, useful to the families in need. For the information to be useful, it must identify not only services that are available, but also services that are accessible. The professional literature[9,13] suggests that the basic information required for the I&R system include organization name, address, telephone number, hours of operation, eligibility requirements (eg, age, gender, income level), services provided, area served, and populations served.[9,13] This information is usually enough to identify available services; however, it may not be enough to assist the caller in accessing those services. Based on the experience in South Carolina, the I&R system for persons with special needs must also include details about the services provided, names of contact people for specific services, information regarding mandates governing organizations, and grievance or due process procedures provided by organizations. For example, Public Law 94-142 guarantees specific services and rights to children with handicaps, including specific due process procedures to protect those rights. It is often not enough to refer parents concerned about their child's education to the local school; when no one else has told the parent the information specialist should be able to effectively inform the parents about their child's rights, and refer them to the contact for special education in the district. If the parent is not satisfied by the services, the I&R should be equipped to provide information to enable the parent to access the due process system.

For parents needing to access the Medicaid system, especially model waivers, it is not enough to refer them to the local Department of Social Services (or its equivalent). The information specialist must also know that the state has waivers, must know the name of the waiver program, and should know the contact person overseeing that specific wavier. These details enable the information specialist to not only refer the caller to available services, but to also assist the caller to access the services.

Classification systems

The organization of the information within any I&R system enhances the usefulness of the information. SCSIS organizes information in three ways: by services provided, conditions and disabilities treated, and geographic area served. Each information taxonomy provides a framework for organization. A key feature is the flexibility to expand this framework. As new services develop or additional conditions are identified, new categories can be added to the existing taxonomies. SCSIS, therefore, grows with the development of community services.

The *services* taxonomy includes approximately 220 categories under which services are classified. The general categories include counseling, diagnosis and evaluation, education, financial assistance, indirect services, medical treatment, residential services, rehabilitation, specialized equipment, and support services.

Descriptions of the services provided are not limited to a category name; organizations can describe specifically how they provide each service.

The *conditions* taxonomy comprises approximately 400 listings, including handicapping conditions such as mental retardation; cerebral palsy; autism; physical disability; hearing, vision, or speech impairment; and Down, Menkes, and Williams syndromes.

The *geographic areas* covered by SCSIS include all the counties in South Carolina because counties conform to the service delivery pattern in South Carolina. The areas covered could also include school districts, health districts, Indian Health Districts, parishes, or other catchment areas appropriate to the service delivery system in other states.

Accessibility to the system

Whether the I&R system is accessible to those who need it depends on two criteria: (1) Do consumers know about the I&R system? (2) If they know about it, can they utilize it?[9,15] Levinson refers to access in terms of "whether those who need help can obtain it."[9(p14)] To ensure that those who need information know about the I&R system, public awareness must be a major focus of the system. Public awareness must be widespread, targeted to specific groups, and continual.

Typically, access to I&R system is by telephone, mail, walk-in, and recently, by direct computer linkage. The model discussed here emphasizes use of a toll-free (1-800) telephone number. Harris and Associates[12] found that 80% of people with disabilities reported that they would use an 800 number to obtain information. This method allows equal access to almost everyone, regardless of income or education level. It also offers the anonymity some families prefer when they begin their search for services.

Trained information specialists

The SCSIS uses paid staff who are trained to assist families of children with disabilities or other special needs. The information specialists, or counselors as they are often called, are the heart and soul of information and referral systems that serve persons with special needs. To provide useful information and appropriate referrals, the information specialist must accurately assess the inquirer's needs and identify the required information or appropriate referrals.

Unless the information specialist accurately assesses the inquirer's needs, appropriate referrals cannot be made. In fact, by failing to determine the caller's needs, the information specialist may add to the caller's frustration by sending him or her to inappropriate agencies. Often, a consumer will request specific services because he or she has heard someone else use the terms; however, the jargon used in human services may complicate communication. The information specialist, therefore, must obtain enough facts about the caller's situation to determine which services will meet his or her needs.

Once the needs are identified, the information specialist must identify appropriate organizations. This requires that the information specialist have a clear understanding of the human service delivery system, that is, how organizations provide services and how consumers access these services. By discussing the available options, the information specialist and the caller decide which providers meet the family's needs, based on such things as cost of services, location of the provider, availability of transportation, etc.

Computer

The computer enables the information specialist to provide information and referral services. The computer stores vast amounts of information about a multitude of resources, and organizes this information so that the specialist can access the needed information quickly. More importantly, the computer enables the specialist to update information so that the most current information is available to all staff.

To fulfill the secondary purpose of a good I&R system, information about requests must be collected and organized to provide aggregate information regarding service needs, gaps, and duplications. The computer plays an important role in identifying service gaps and reporting the level of service requests to policy planners. It enables the information specialist, during the course of the call, to document information about the caller (ie, age, gender, area of residence, disability/handicapping condition, service needs, etc.) and about referrals made. This information is stored in the computer. The SCSIS provides monthly reports summarizing these data to the Developmental Disabilities Council to assist in planning for service delivery in South Carolina.

SCSIS operates on IBM personal computers connected by a local area network (LAN). The software and training materials were developed by the Center for Developmental Disabilities and the Computer Services Division at The University of South Carolina. This totally integrated system uses a combination of commercial and in-house software to enter and retrieve information, document caller requests, word process, and track agencies contacted for data collection or update and reporting automatically.

Other states using this model

Currently, Louisiana, New Mexico, and Oklahoma are using the software developed in South Carolina and the SCSIS model to provide statewide information and referral for persons with disabilities. Agencies administering these programs vary from state to state and include developmental disabilities councils, protection and advocacy systems, university-affiliated programs, health departments and children's hospitals. As of this writing, both South Carolina and Louisiana are adapting their existing system to meet the needs of the central directory requirement of Public Law 99-457. Staff of the Lead Agency in Hawaii has also decided to use this model as the central directory for that state.

IMPLICATIONS FOR PUBLIC LAW 99-457

Whether developing a new system or adapting an existing one, several practical issues must be considered in order to address the specific requirements of a central directory of resources for infants and toddlers with handicaps. These authors recommend that an advisory board guide the development of this system. South Carolina established a "panel of experts" composed of an early intervention specialist, a developmental pediatrician, a neonatal intensive care unit nurse, parents of infants and toddlers with disabilities, and other professionals knowledgeable about the special needs of infants with disabilities and their families. While this panel had no direct authority over the system, the members acted in an advisory capacity and oversaw the expansion of this system to meet the needs of infants and toddlers with disabilities and their families. The panel provided input on all major activities. For example, the panel assisted in the review and modification of the content of the system, which included the addition of service categories and handicapping conditions to the taxonomies. They also assisted in developing individualized questionnaires for specialized practitioners and provided training for the information specialists. Other major issues, related to the five major components of an I&R system and how South Carolina has adapted SCSIS, are described below.

Database of information and resources

Public Law 99-457 requires that the central directory include early intervention services, resources and experts available, and research and demonstration projects. The major challenge in developing the information database is not in identifying appropriate providers to include, but rather in understanding what a family needs to know about specific providers. For example, to know that a physician will treat an infant with Werdnig-Hoffman's disease is only part of the information; what is more important to the family is to identify a physician who will provide "care management" for a child with this disability and monitor and treat the child's condition over an extended period of time. Each group of experts and individual providers has unique characteristics. To capture this "additional" information, the SCSIS staff developed separate data collection questionnaires for individual providers (eg, physicians, speech/language therapists, physical and occupational therapists, and day care providers).

Other significant changes or additions to the information database include expansion of data on relevant legislation (ie, relating to parent's and child's rights), the service delivery system (how programs interact or work together), and what the limits to services are. A key consideration for parents of infants with disabilities is their need to link with other parents; therefore, SCSIS includes a parent-to-parent registry to link parents of children having similar disabilities. As with all providers included in an I&R system, the competence and quality of services must be addressed. In the case of the parent-to-parent registry, only parents completing appropriate training are included in the system.

Classification systems

For the information in the I&R system to address the needs of specific groups with special needs and for it to be organized effectively for ease in reporting, each classification schema must include categories specific to the needs of the specific groups of people. The SCSIS staff expanded both the services and conditions taxonomies to accommodate specificities of infants and toddlers. Approximately 20 service categories were added to that taxonomy, and approximately 15 conditions were added to the conditions taxonomy (eg, bronchopulmonary dysplasia, cytomegalovirus, deglutition disorders, failure to thrive).

Accessibility to the I&R system

Many families with premature, low-birth-weight, or otherwise at risk infants are low income families. Access to information must be affordable; for these families, that means free. The use of the toll-free telephone line will ensure direct access to information for families and for the professionals who serve them. Efforts to publicize the central directory should target both families and professionals and should be widespread and routine. Strategies should include, but not be limited to, the following:

1. Develop appropriate printed and other materials (including a brochure or flyer targeting families, 10 or 30 second video or audio public service announcements).
2. Target specific groups most likely to serve infants and toddlers (eg, health department clinics, pediatric and neonatal nurses, developmental clinics, schools, day care centers, parent groups).
3. Inform the general public.

Since parents of infants and toddlers with handicaps are less likely to be connected to formal groups, it is crucial to find ways to reach individual parents. Most television and radio stations, as well as newspapers (especially in rural communities), are willing to run public service announcements. Utility companies and water services may be willing to include inserts in monthly mailings. Given the diversity of the educational, intellectual, and economic levels of these families, all available public awareness techniques should be used.

Training for information specialists

Because of the nature of this population (parents of infants and toddlers with handicaps), the information specialists must work as "problem solvers." Two problems they face are identifying service needs when there is no diagnosis, and identifying early intervention services as they become available. Since most states are just developing systems of care for early intervention, the information specialists must maximize the use of existing programs and stay up-to-date on the developing services. Training issues include developing a greater understanding of early childhood handicapping conditions; learning which delays suggest needs for services; and learning how services, and access to services, differ for very young children (eg, exceptions to eligibility criteria). In South Carolina, the panel of experts has provided training in the above listed areas.

Computer

Given the evolving nature of the system of care for early intervention in most states, the computer plays an important role in enabling the information specialist to stay up-to-date on services. As new services are developed, information about them can be added to the central directory and made readily available to the information specialists.

For the central directory to be used effectively as a planning tool for service development and implementation, it must be able to document requests for information, identified needs, services available, and gaps in services. With the SCSIS model, information is automatically documented so that reports can be generated easily to calculate requests for specific services (eg, early intervention services, respite care, financial assistance) in specified geographic areas.

BENEFITS

The system described in this paper provides a model computer-based information and referral system with specific applications for use as the central directory required by Public Law 99-457. This model, which blends features such as toll-free access, trained information specialists, and a computer-driven database, offers benefits to families, professionals, and planners. It provides a personal touch when used to assist families to meet their needs and offers families the options and information they need to face everyday challenges. The flexibility of the system allows it to grow with the changing service delivery system as services and new systems of care evolve.

To maximize the use and impact of the central directory, it should be integrated with other components of Public Law 99-457, such as Child Find, the Unduplicated Count, and the Case Management System. The central directory offers a tool for identifying infants and toddlers with special needs and it can function as a feeder to the case management system for a coordinated system of care for infants and toddlers. This integration can simply coordinate referrals between the components or centralize entry into the system through one point. At this time, South Carolina has chosen to coordinate referrals among the components. The toll-free number for the Central Directory will be publicized on all public awareness materials for Public law 99-457 as the central number for information. The information specialists will then refer the callers to the appropriate resource in their own county.

• • •

Each state has its own systems and structures in place within which it must work to implement the mandates of Public Law 99-457. Models such as the one described in this article are tools available to create a coordinated system of early intervention services. The effectiveness of those systems, however, will be determined by a state's ability to use appropriate tools within the structure of its system of care.

REFERENCES

1. Turnbull AP, Turnbull, HR. *Families, professionals, and exceptionality.* Columbus, Oh. Charles E. Merrill; 1986.
2. Public Law 99-457, Part H: Education for All Handicapped Children Act 1987, Section 676 (b) (7), p1146.
3. Silverstein R. *A Window of Opportunity, PL99-457, the Intent and Spirit of PL99-457: A Sourcebook.* Washington, DC: National Center for Clinical Infant Programs; 1986.
4. Hobbs N, Perrin JM, Ireys, HT. *Summary of Findings and Recommendations of Public Policies Affecting Chronically Ill Children and Their Families.* Center for the Study of Families and Children. Nashville, TN; Vanderbilt Institute for Public Policy Studies; 1983.
5. Shelton TL, Jeppson ES, Johnson BH. *Family-Centered Care for Children with Special Health Care Needs.* Washington, DC: Association for the Care of Children's Health; 1987.
6. Dunst CJ, Trivette CM. Enabling and empowering families: Conceptual and intervention issues. *Sch Psych Rev.* 1987;16:443–456.
7. Rappaport J. Terms of empowerment/Exemplars of prevention: toward a theory for community psychology. *Am J Community Psychol* 1987;15:121–128.
8. Mayfield KL, Wiles DL. Computerized Information and Referral: A Resource for You. In: *1988 Proceedings: Empowering Families for Better Health.* Columbia, SC: University Printing; 1988.

9. Levinson RW. Information and Referral Services. In: Gilbert N, Specht H, eds. Handbook of the Social Services. Englewood Cliffs, NJ: Prentice-Hall; 1981:13–34.
10. United Way of America. *National Standards for Information and Referral.* Alexandria, VA: United Way of America; 1983.
11. Morris R. What lies ahead for I&R services. *Journal of the Alliance of Information and Referral Systems.* 1987;9:25–32.
12. Harris L. and Associates, Inc. *Disabled Americans' Self Perceptions: Bringing Disabled Americans into the Mainstream.* New York, New York: International Center for the Disabled, Study No. 854009, 1986.
13. Bailey DB, Simeonsson RJ. Assessing Needs of Families with Handicapped Infants. *J Special Educ.* 1988;22:117–127.
14. Henry AC. The importance of resource files in information and referral delivery. *J All I R Sys.* 1987;8:39–47.
15. Downey NA, Castellani PJ, Tausig MB. The provision of information and referral services in the community. *Ment Retardation.* 1985;23:21–25.

Gastrostomies: Indications, management, and weaning

Christy L.A. Nelson, MS, OTR
Department of Occupational Therapy
Glenrose Rehabilitation Hospital
Assistant Professor
Department of Occupational Therapy
Faculty of Rehabilitation Medicine
The University of Alberta

Robert A. Hallgren, MD, FACS
Department of Surgery
Royal Alexandra General Hospital
Associate Clinical Professor
Faculty of Surgery
The University of Alberta
Edmonton, Alberta, Canada

GASTROSTOMY placement is becoming increasingly common in children with developmental disabilities. At first, management of the gastrostomy may appear to be quite complex. However, with an understanding of the techniques and principles involved, those working with children with gastrostomies can implement a feeding plan that is beneficial to health and development.

INDICATIONS

The child who requires nonoral enteral nutrition for three months or longer is considered a candidate for gastrostomy tube placement.[1] Alimentary anomalies, chronic disease, central nervous system (CNS) disorders, and developmental limitations are conditions that can hinder feeding enough to necessitate gastrostomy surgery.[2–8]

Alimentary anomalies

Structural anomalies of the mouth, esophagus, and bowel all potentially result in long-term dependence on nonoral nutrition. Micrognathia (a small receding jaw) often leads to the need for nonoral nutrition in the newborn if the micrognathia is severe. The limited size of the oral cavity prevents nippling and can lead to respiratory compromise during feeding. Micrognathia and other oral malformations are common features in syndromes such as Pierre Robin syndrome, Nager-Reynier syndrome, and Goldenhar's syndrome.

Anomalies of the esophagus, such as esophageal cleft, fistula, stricture, and atresia, can result in gastrostomy tube placement in infants shortly after birth. Risk of aspiration in infants with esophageal cleft or fistula and inability of formula to reach the stomach in infants with stricture or atresia can lead to total dependence on nonoral nutrition until the conditions are surgically corrected.

Anomalies and diseases of the bowel often lead to the need for parenteral nutrition (nutrition provided directly into the bloodstream) due to the inability of the bowel to adequately digest and absorb nutrients. Children who are dependent on

The authors acknowledge Susan Crack for her artistic assistance.

Inf Young Children 1989; 2(1): 66–74

parenteral nutrition for long periods of time can be resistant to reinstating oral feeding after the bowel problems have resolved.[9,10] If this resistance cannot be overcome, then the children may receive a gastrostomy for long-term nutritional management. Bowel conditions that may lead to gastrostomy placement include necrotizing enterocolitis, short bowel syndrome, omphalocele, bowel obstruction, malrotation, and atresia.

Chronic disease

Weakness, lethargy, and anorexia are common findings in children with serious illnesses such as renal, pulmonary, cardiac, and hepatic diseases. The child's state, as well as special nutritional needs caused by the disease, can lead to the need for supplemental nutritional support by IV or nasogastric tube. If these interventions are needed for long periods of time, the child may become dependent on this type of nutritional support, leading to the need for gastrostomy surgery as a solution for long-term nutritional care.

CNS disorders

Neuromuscular involvement of the oral and pharyngeal musculature can hinder oral feeding to the point that long-term nonoral nourishment is necessary. Poor oral motor control can result in excessively long mealtimes and inadequate quantity of intake. Increased susceptibility to illness is likely to be the result of long-term malnutrition. If the oral feeding problems do not improve, then gastrostomy placement may be necessary in order to prevent chronic health problems.

Significant neuromuscular involvement of the pharynx can lead to aspiration of foods and fluids into the lungs. If the aspiration is severe or chronic, then oral feeding may need to be restricted in order to protect the health and life of the child.

CNS disorders that may lead to gastrostomy placement include cerebral palsy, postinfectious encephalopathies (cytomegalovirus, herpes, meningitis), posttraumatic encephalopathies (near drowning, head trauma, near-miss sudden infant death syndrome), degenerative diseases, impaired brain growth and brain anomalies (microcephaly, holoprosencephaly, anencephaly), and brain tumors.

Developmental limitations

Some children with mental retardation appear to have atypical hunger and thirst drives. No apparent medical reason can be found for their lack of desire to eat and drink. Chronic undernutrition can lead to anorexia, which further complicates the situation. Some of these children respond quite poorly to oral feeding therapy and subsequently need gastrostomy surgery.

GASTROSTOMY SURGERIES

A gastrostomy is a surgically created fistula between the stomach and the skin. This fistula is usually made midway between the navel and the left nipple (Fig 1). A gastrostomy tube (also called a gastrostomy catheter) is placed in that fistula so that feedings can be administered. Gastrostomy catheters are not permanently sutured to the stomach or the skin. Therefore, the catheters can be removed from the fistula without trauma.

Gastrostomy surgeries can be performed under either general or local anesthesia. A variety of surgical procedures have been described for forming the gastrostomy fistula.[11–18] The numerous types of surgeries (and surgery variations) indicate the difficulty of creating a completely satisfactory communication between the stomach and the abdominal surface. Two techniques are commonly employed for pediatric patients: gastrostomies with indwelling catheters (the Stamm and percutaneous endoscopic gastrostomy) and gastrostomies without indwelling catheters (gastric tubes).

Gastrostomies with indwelling catheters

The Stamm procedure forms a serosal fistula between the stomach and the abdominal surface. A serosal fistula is an opening that is lined with serous membrane

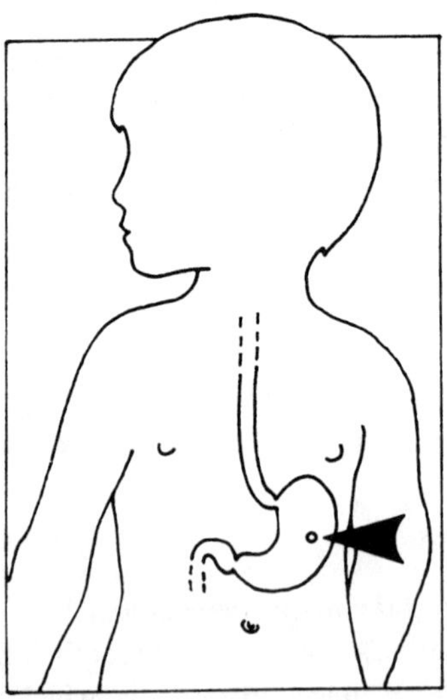

Fig 1. The surgically created gastrostomy fistula is usually placed midway between the navel and the left nipple (arrowhead).

(the membrane that covers the abdominal cavity). This fistula is formed by making a small opening in the abdomen and placing a gastrostomy catheter in the opening, which inverts the stomach wall and forms a serosal tube around the gastrostomy tube. The gastrostomy catheter is drawn through this opening through a separate incision. Children who have had a Stamm procedure will therefore have a surgical incision in addition to the gastrostomy fistula.

The percutaneous endoscopic gastrostomy (PEG) is performed with the use of a gastroscope. The gastroscope is placed into the stomach through the mouth and esophagus. This gastroscope secures a long suture that has been placed in the stomach by way of a small hole in the abdominal wall made by a sharp trocar. This suture is pulled through the abdominal wall, stomach, and esophagus and then out of the mouth; the result is a thread that runs from the exterior of the abdomen (through the stomach and esophagus) to the exterior of the mouth. At this point, a gastrostomy catheter is attached to the suture and is pulled through the mouth, esophagus, stomach, and out of the abdominal wall. The tube is secured in place by internal and external cross bars.

Once the fistula is formed by either of these methods, it is important that the gastrostomy catheter remain in place. If removed, the gastrostomy opening will rapidly close, making replacement of the catheter difficult. If the catheter has been removed for an extended period of time, dilation of the fistula may be necessary before the catheter can be reinserted. If the child no longer requires the gastrostomy, the catheter can be removed, and the fistula will close naturally.

Gastrostomies without indwelling catheters

A gastric tube is a type of fistula that is lined with the mucosa of the stomach. Gastric tube surgery (the Janeway and Beck-Jianu) forms a permanent opening (or stoma) that allows for intermittent insertion of a catheter for feeding. Since this opening is permanent, the gastrostomy catheter does not need to remain in place. If the child no longer needs the gastrostomy, surgery is required in order to close the fistula.

GASTROSTOMY MANAGEMENT

Following surgery, guidelines are developed to assist the family with gastrostomy management at home. These management plans often address type of gastrostomy catheter to be used, guidelines for formula preparation, method of gavage, and techniques for stoma and catheter care.

Types of gastrostomy catheters

The de Pezzer, Malecot, and Foley are common types of gastrostomy catheters (Fig 2). The de Pezzer is a slender tube approximately 14 in long with a protuber-

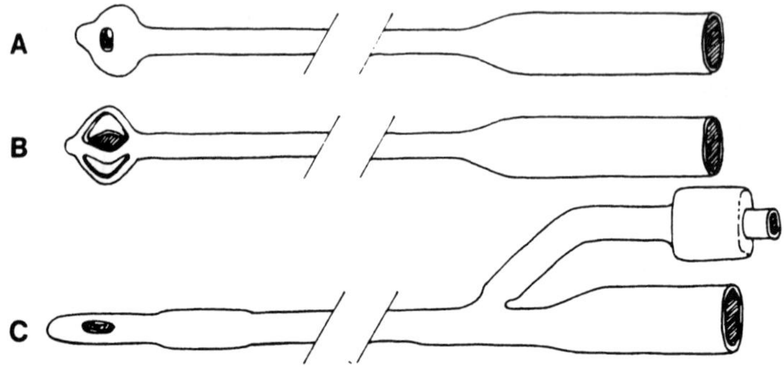

Fig 2. Gastrostomy catheters—(**A**) de Pezzer; (**B**) Malecot; and (**C**) Foley.

ance on one end. This protuberance is firm and has two small holes, The firmness of the bulb aids in maintaining the catheter's placement in the interior of the stomach. When in the correct position, the bulb should be snug against the interior stomach wall (Fig 3). The tendency for this catheter to maintain its position in the stomach makes it the preferred gastrostomy catheter by some.[5] Others have found the holes too small and have recommended modifications to the de Pezzer.[6,19] Families have found this tube easy to use but difficult to replace at home due to the firmness of the bulb.

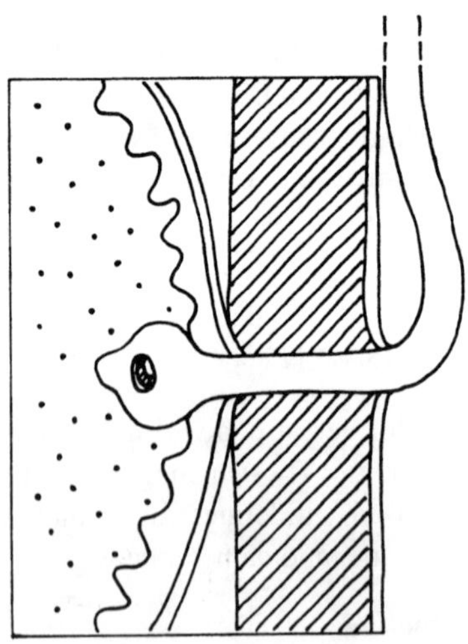

Fig 3. When the gastrostomy catheter is in the correct position, the bulb should be snug against the interior stomach wall.

The Malecot has a softer bulb that looks like an open basket. This soft basket allows easy placement of the catheter and quick passage of nutrients through the tube. However, the tube must be securely anchored in order to maintain the flexible basket in position against the interior stomach wall.

The Foley catheter is approximately 17 in long with an inflatable balloon on one end and a bifid canal on the other. When deflated, the tube can be easily placed into the gastrostomy stoma. Inflation of the balloon (by instilling water into the bifid canal via syringe) holds the catheter in place (Fig 4). The ease of placement of the Foley makes it attractive for families to use as a replacement catheter at home if the original tube is inadvertently removed. However, there are some disadvantages to the Foley. The balloons are fragile and may burst if grainy foods or medications are administered. Also, esophageal obstruction with rupture[2,20] and gastric outlet obstruction with duodenal perforation[21] due to gastrostomy tube migration have been reported.

Gauderer, Picha, and Izant[22] described a new device for nonoral feeding—the gastrostomy "button." This skin-level device is placed in an existing gastrostomy site. The button has a one-way valve that prevents leakage of stomach contents out of the stoma. The button is intended to be used as a substitute for traditional gastrostomy catheters. A feeding catheter is used only to administer formula and is removed when the feeding is complete.[23] Replacing the indwelling tube with a temporary catheter that is used only during feeding makes this feeding method attractive to many families. One disadvantage is that the child must not be active during the feeding, or the catheter may become disconnected.[23]

Formulas

Type and volume of formula given depend on the child's age and size, current medical condition, history of allergies or intolerances, and degree of gastrointestinal function. A variety of commercially prepared formulas is available to meet the

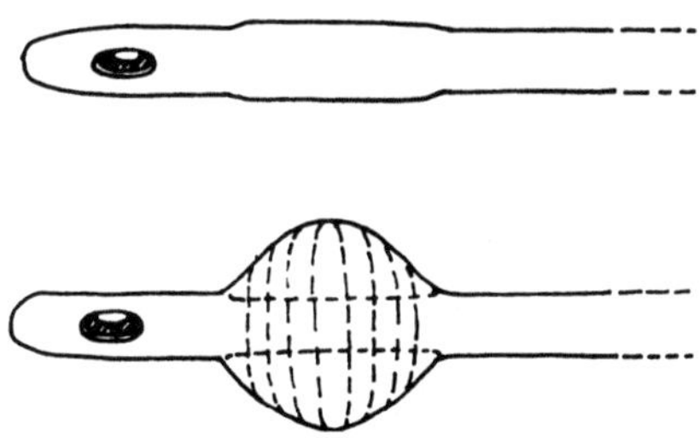

Fig 4. The Foley gastrostomy catheter with balloon deflated (top) and inflated (bottom).

needs of the tube-nourished child (Table 1); however, home-prepared formulas, as recommended by dietitians, can also be used. A number of factors need to be considered when choosing a commercially prepared or a home-prepared formula[1]: dietary needs for nutrients, fluids, and fiber (numerous commercially prepared formulas are available to meet specific dietary needs); cost (commercially prepared formulas are more expensive than home-prepared formulas); preparation time (home-prepared formulas can be more time consuming); preparation method (home blenders may not puree foods adequately for administration through the slender catheter); sanitation (home-prepared formulas have a greater risk for bacterial contamination); and family preference.

Since the growing child's needs for calories, protein, carbohydrates, fat, vitamins, minerals, and trace elements change over time, formula quantity and composition should be periodically reviewed by a nutritionist.

Table 1. Commercially prepared formulas

Classification	*Product*	*Manufacturer*	*Uses*
Milk based	Enfamil Similac SMA Milumil	Mead Johnson Ross Wyeth Milupa	Formula for infants
Soy based	Isomil Neo-Mull Soy Nursoy ProSobee Soyalac	Ross Syntex Wyeth Mead Johnson Loma Linda	Formula for infants sensitive to cow milk or lactose
Protein modified	Nutramigen Pregestimil RCF	Mead Johnson Mead Johnson Ross	Formulas for infants who have sensitivity to cow milk, sensitivity to soy protein, severe diarrhea, or malabsorption
Fat modified	Portagen	Mead Johnson	Formulas for infants and children who have poor digestion or malabsorption of long chain fatty acids
Lactose free	Ensure Ensure Plus	Ross Ross	Formulas for children who have lactose intolerance
Isotonic	Compleat Modified Isocal Isocal HN Osmolite Osmolite HN	Sandoz Mead Johnson Mead Johnson Ross Ross	Formulas for children who are intolerant of formula with high osmolality (formulas that are hypertonic)
High fiber	Compleat B Compleat Modified Enrich	Sandoz Sandoz Ross	Formulas for children who require formula with fiber

Gavage methods

Prior to beginning the feeding, the placement of the tube should be checked, stomach contents aspirated, and adjustments made to the feeding as appropriate based on the amount of residual volume in the stomach.[24–26] To begin the feeding, the gastrostomy tube is connected to a feeding bag or a 60 mL syringe. The rate of fluid flow can be controlled by hand, gravity, or mechanical pump.

In hand-controlled feeding, a 60 mL syringe must be used. The fluid is placed in the syringe and is pushed down into the gastrostomy tube via a bulb or syringe plunger. Administration of the feeding is usually completed within minutes. The quickness of the feeding makes this method attractive to many families; however, these feedings are not always tolerated by pediatric patients. Gagging, nausea, and vomiting are common problems associated with this method.

Gravity-controlled feeding is better tolerated by many children. In gravity-controlled feeding, the fluid is placed in the syringe or bag and flows into the gastrostomy tube by gravity. The rate of the flow is controlled by elevating (faster rate) or lowering (slower rate) the feeding bag. Gravity-controlled feeding is usually completed in approximately 30 minutes.

Continuous-drip feedings can be used for children who cannot tolerate large volumes of formula given at one time. The rate of fluid flow is controlled by a mechanical pump designed for tube feedings; a variety of pumps is available for use with pediatric patients.[1] The rate of fluid flow may range from a few mL to 300 mL per hour and may be given over a 24-hour period. However, feedings over 24 hours can significantly limit the child's activity. Therefore, continuous infusion is often given at night and supplemented by small bolus feedings during the day if tolerated by the child. Continuous-infusion feedings have been reported to be beneficial to children with intestinal disease[27] and complex congenital heart disease.[28] However, this method of feeding has been reported to interfere with absorption of the seizure medication phenytoin.[29]

Stoma and catheter care

The gastrostomy stoma should be inspected daily for signs of leakage, bleeding, and skin irritation. Daily cleansing of the area with soap and water is recommended.[25] In addition, silver nitrate applications may be needed to control granulation tissue that may form around the gastrostomy opening.

Even though there is not a specific schedule for changing the gastrostomy tube, the catheter will need to be periodically replaced due to inadvertent removal or tube deterioration. Correct placement and secure anchoring of the new catheter are quite important in order to minimize complications due to tube migration. Gastrostomy tube changing and anchoring techniques have been described by several authors.[19,25,26,30]

PROBLEMS

Problems seen in children requiring gastrostomy surgery include gastroesophageal reflux, formula intolerance, and problems related to stoma and catheter care.

Gastroesophageal reflux

Gastroesophageal reflux (GER) is the regurgitation of stomach contents back into the esophagus. Aspiration and failure to thrive can be the result of untreated GER. GER is a common problem in children with severe mental retardation.[31] Also, neurologically involved patients have been reported to have a high incidence of GER following gastrostomy surgery.[32] If the reflux is severe, or does not respond to medical intervention, then antireflux surgery may be needed at the time of gastrostomy placement or at some point after the gastrostomy surgery.

The Nissen fundoplication is one type of antireflux surgery. The Nissen fundoplication decreases the possibility of reflux by wrapping the fundus of the stomach around the lower esophagus. This exerts external pressure on the lower esophagus and, as a result, improves the function of the lower esophageal sphincter. This procedure is increasingly performed in patients with permanent gastrostomies to prevent the significant complication of aspiration pneumonia. As a result, it is often performed at the time of gastrostomy creation.

Formula intolerance

Symptoms of formula intolerance include abdominal cramping, diarrhea, and vomiting. These symptoms may be caused by food allergies, lactose intolerance, hypertonic formula, contaminated formula, or improper administration of the feeding.

Cramping, diarrhea, and vomiting can be caused by an allergy to the protein in the formula. Children can show allergies to cow milk protein, soy protein, or both. Changing the source of the protein or use of a protein-modified formula (see Table 1) can alleviate the symptoms.

Lactose is a disaccharide (carbohydrate) found in milk-based formulas. Infants who are lactose intolerant exhibit signs of gastrointestinal distress shortly after the feeding. Use of a lactose-free formula (see Table 1) alleviates the symptoms.

Formulas that are hypertonic can also cause distress in children. Hypertonic formulas (formulas that are more concentrated than body plasma) draw water into the gastrointestinal tract, which can lead to diarrhea.[24] Addition of medications to feedings has been found to contribute to the hypertonic properties of formulas.[33] Isotonic formulas (formulas that have the same concentration as plasma) can alleviate the gastrointestinal problems caused by those that are hypertonic. Isotonic formulas are listed in Table 1.

Bacterial contamination has been reported in home-prepared formulas[1] and in formulas administered via continuous infusion.[34] Home-prepared formulas require refrigeration and should be used within 24 hours. Commercially prepared formulas require refrigeration after opening and should be used within 48 hours. Formulas administered by continuous infusion should not be exposed to room air for more than four to eight hours.[1]

Formula administered too quickly[1] and formula that is too cold when given[35] have been shown to cause gastrointestinal distress in tube-nourished patients. These problems can be alleviated by modifying the feeding technique.

Stoma care

Infection, skin irritation, and leakage of gastric contents are problems related to the stoma. Stoma leakage has been reported to be a greater problem in children than adults due to the thinner abdominal wall, excess motion of the tube, increased intraabdominal pressure from crying, and large volume of feeding as compared to stomach size.[36] The metabolic imbalance caused by excessive or chronic loss of gastric electrolytes can be a serious threat to health and life.[2,37] Medical attention is recommended for stoma-related problems.

Catheter care

Gastrostomy catheter migration is a well-known problem in pediatric patients.[2,5,6,20,21,38–40] Nausea, vomiting, and diarrhea have been reported as well as gastrointestinal obstruction and perforation. Conscientious checking of tube placement and secure anchoring of the catheter are critical in order to minimize problems related to catheter migration.

REINSTATING ORAL FEEDING

Children who have been nourished via nonoral methods for long periods of time often have difficulty returning to oral feeding. This difficulty may be due to lack of oral feeding experience, poor oral motor control, medical conditions, or behavioral resistance. Reinstating oral feeding can be a very complex and often time-consuming process that is overwhelming for many families. A variety of approaches have been described to assist the tube-nourished child in developing oral feeding skills to the point that gastrostomy feedings can be discontinued.[7–10,41–44] Extensive description of these approaches is beyond the scope of this article.

Prior to removing the gastrostomy tube, the child must be able to swallow safely without aspiration, eat comfortably without excessive effort or fatigue, and consume foods and fluids in amounts adequate for promoting growth and health.

• • •

Feeding by gastrostomy is becoming increasingly common in children with developmental disabilities. The problems that have been reported in children with gastrostomies can be minimized with careful monitoring and management of the stoma, catheter, and feeding process. Fortunately, gastrostomy and Nissen fundoplication surgeries do not preclude oral feeding ability. Oral feeding can continue immediately after gastrostomy placement (if the child's medical condition allows) or can be reinstated at a later time.

Gastrostomy feeding can be a safe method of providing nourishment to children who are not capable of consuming adequate nutrition by oral means. A well-defined feeding management plan that includes ongoing support to the family can lead to a feeding regimen that is pleasant for both caretaker and child.

REFERENCES

1. Moore MC, Greene HL: Tube feeding of infants and children. *Pediatr Clin North Am* 1985;32:401–417.
2. Holder TM, Gross RE: Temporary gastrostomy in pediatric surgery: Experience with 187 cases. *Pediatrics* 1960;26:36–41.
3. Haws EB, Sieber WK, Kiesewetter WB: Complications of tube gastrostomy in infants and children. *Ann Surg* 1966;2:284–290.
4. Parrish RA, Cohen J: Temporary tube gastrostomy. *Am Surg* 1972;38:168–171.
5. Gallagher MW, Tyson KRT, Ashcraft KW: Gastrostomy in pediatric patients: An analysis of complications and techniques. *Surgery* 1973;74:536–539.
6. Campbell JR, Sasaki TM: Gastrostomy in infants and children: Analysis of complications and techniques. *Am Surg* 1974;40:505–508.
7. Blackman JA, Nelson CLA: Reinstituting oral feeding in children fed by gastrostomy tube. *Clin Pediatr* 1985;24:434–438.
8. Blackman JA, Nelson CLA: Rapid introduction of oral feedings to tube-fed patients. *J Dev Behav Pediatr* 1987;8:63–67.
9. Geertsma MA, Hyams JS, Pelletier JM, et al: Feeding resistance after parenteral hyperalimentation. *Am J Dis Child* 1985;139:255–256.
10. Handen BL, Mandell FM, Russo DC: Feeding induction in children who refuse to eat. *Am J Dis Child* 1986;140:52–54.
11. Stamm M: Gastrostomy by a new method. *Med News* 1984;65:234.
12. Dragstedt LR, Haymond HE, Ellis JC: Cannula gastrostomy and enterostomy. *Surg Gynecol Obstet* 1933;56:799–801.
13. Glassman JA: A new aseptic double-valved tubogastrostomy. *Surg Gynecol Obstet* 1939;68:789–791.
14. Pourfar M, Chafiian J: Permanent gastrostomy in severely brain-damaged children. *Dev Med Child Neurol* 1969;11:214–217.

15. Thomas CG, Croom RD: A method for temporary gastrostoma. *Surg Gynecol Obstet* 1970;131:292–294.
16. Preshaw RM: Percutaneous method for inserting a feeding gastrostomy tube. *Surg Gynecol Obstet* 1981;152:659–660.
17. McGovern B: Janeway gastrostomy in children with CP. *J Pediatr Surg* 1984;19:800–802.
18. Larson DE, Burton DD, Schroeder KW, et al: Percutaneous endoscopic gastrostomy: Indications, success, complications, and mortality in 314 consecutive patients. *Gastroenterology* 1987;93:48–52.
19. Paalberg J, Balint JP: Gastrostomy tubes: Practical guidelines for home care. *Pediatr Nurs* 1985;11:99–102.
20. Frech RS, Roper C, McAlister WH: Esophageal rupture secondary to pyloric obstruction by a gastrostomy Foley catheter balloon. *J Can Assoc Radiol* 1970;21:262–265.
21. Ballinger WF, McLaughlin ED, Baranski EJ: Jeunal overlay closure of duodenum in the newborn: Lateral duodenal tear caused by gastrostomy tube. *Surgery* 1966;59:450–454.
22. Gauderer MWL, Picha GJ, Izant RJ: The gastrostomy "button": A simple, skin-level nonrefluxing device for long–term enteral feedings. *J Pediatr Surg* 1984;19:803–805.
23. Huth MM, O'Brien ME: The gastrostomy feeding button. *Pediatr Nurs* 1987;13:241–246.
24. Konstantinides NN, Shronts E: Tube feeding: Managing the basics. *Am J Nurs* 1983;83:1312–1320.
25. Perez RC, Bechom L, Jebara L, et al: Care of the child with a gastrostomy tube: Common and practical concerns. *Issues Compr Nurs* 1984;7:107–119.
26. Zechman RAD, Ross A, Watkins J: *Pediatric Adaptive Technologies: Gastrostomy Tube Feeding* (videotape). Seattle, University of Washington, 1985.
27. Parker P, Stroop S, Greene H: A controlled comparison of continuous feeding in the treatment of infants with intestinal disease. *J Pediatr* 1981;99:360–364.
28. Vanderhoof JA, Hofschire PJ, Baluff MA, et al: Continuous enteral feedings: An important adjunct to the management of complex congenital heart disease. *Am J Dis Child* 1982;136:825–827.
29. Bauer LA: Interference of oral phenytoin absorption by continuous drip nasogastric feedings. *Neurology* 1982;32:570–572.
30. Kappel DA, Leape LL: A method for gastrostomy fixation. *J Pediatr Surg* 1975;10:523–524.
31. Sondheimer JM, Morris BA: Gastroesophageal reflux among severely retarded children. *J Pediatr* 1979;94:710–714.
32. Mollitt DL, Golladay ES, Seibert JJ: Symptomatic gastroesophageal reflux following gastrostomy in neurologically impaired patients. *Pediatrics* 1985;75:1124–1126.
33. White KC, Harkavy KL: Hypertonic formula resulting from added oral medications. *Am J Dis Child* 1982;136:931–933.
34. Hostetler C, Lipman TO, Geraghty M, et al: Bacterial safety of reconstituted continuous drip tube feeding. *JPEN* 1982;6:232–235.
35. Kagawa-Busby KS, Heitkemper MM, Hansen BC, et al: Effects of diet temperature on tolerance of enteral feedings. *Nurs Res* 1980;20:276–280.
36. Gauderer MWL, Stellato TA: *Gastrostomies: Evolution, Techniques, Indications, and Complications.* Chicago, Year Book, 1986.
37. Connar RG, Sealy WC: Gastrostomy and its complications. *Ann Surg* 1956;143:245–250.
38. Sherman ML, Cosgrove MJ, Dennis JM: Gastrostomy tube migration. *Am Surg* 1973;39:122–123.

39. Currarino G, Votteler T: Prolapse of the gastrostomy catheter in children. *Am J Roentgenol Radium Ther Nucl Med* 1975;123:737–741.

40. Vade A, Jafri SZH, Agha FP, et al: Radiologic evaluation of gastrostomy complications. *Am J Roentgenol* 1983;141:315–330.

41. Di Scipio WJ, Kaslon K, Ruben RJ: Traumatically acquired conditioned dysphagia in children. *Ann Otol* 1978;87:509–514.

42. Van Dyke DC, Mackay L, Ziaylek EN: Management of severe feeding dysfunction in children with fetal alcohol syndrome. *Clin Pediatr* 1982;21:336–339.

43. Nelson CLA, Blackman JA: *Management of the Child Fed Via Gastrostomy Tube* (videotape). Iowa City, Division of Developmental Disabilities, University of Iowa, 1983.

44. Riordan MM, Iwata BA, Finney JW, et al: Behavioral assessment and treatment of chronic food refusal in handicapped children. *J Appl Behav Anal* 1984;17:327–341.

The new genetics, developmental disabilities, and early intervention

Don C. Van Dyke, MD
Assistant Professor of Pediatrics

Deborah C. Lin-Dyken, MD
Associate in Pediatrics
University Hospital School
Department of Pediatrics
University of Iowa Hospitals and Clinics
Iowa City, Iowa

ALMOST FOUR decades ago, with the discovery of *DNA** as the memory bank of human cells, the field of molecular genetics moved to the forefront of medical and biologic research. The discovery of the structure of DNA and its role as the carrier of genetic information was only the first step. Important discoveries followed with the understanding of coding *sequences* and how genetic information is precisely copied and passed on from cell to cell. The determination of highly specific sequences of *nucleotides* and their translation into *proteins* by means of the molecular machinery of cells was the beginning of our understanding of the data bank of the cell and the regulatory properties of DNA. This knowledge was necessary to bring genetics from the plants of Mendel to our present day understanding of the molecular genetics of disorders such as cystic fibrosis and muscular dystrophy. Before this time, genetics was largely clinical, statistical, and microscopic. Constellations of physical findings called syndromes, abnormalities of growth called dysmorphology, and family pedigrees were the tools of the clinical geneticist. We have gone from the identification of the bands of the *chromosome* to the determination of the sequence of molecules of chromosomal DNA. Our understanding of specific abnormalities in the basic molecular code has allowed us to understand changes in protein structure and function that have broadened our understanding of the biochemical and anatomic changes that result in observed clinical and physiologic findings.

The technology of the last 15 years has produced a rapid escalation of knowledge. Trickles of information have grown into a deluge of findings, flowing together to create an ocean of data.[1–3] The pace has quickened on every level, but particularly at the national and international levels with the initiation of the *Human Genome Project* 2½ years ago.[4] This ambitious project will span the next 15 years and will require an estimated $3 billion to map all areas of the 23 pairs of human chromosomes.[4]

Finding *mutations* (alterations in DNA), such as those that define cystic fibrosis and Duchenne's muscular dystrophy, as was done in the late 1980s, is like trying

We gratefully acknowledge Ginny Miller for her technical and editorial expertise and Susan Eberly, MA, Alfred Healy, MD, Louise Greenswag, RN, PhD, Debora Downey, MA, and Randell Alexander, MD, PhD, for reviewing this manuscript.

**Words appearing in italics are defined in the glossary at the end of this article.*

Inf Young Children 1993; 5(4): 8–19

to find a diamond ring lost in the trash of New York City's landfill.[4,5] The rapid accumulation of new information is due to a number of key technologic breakthroughs in the last 15 years.[1,3] The new technology that led to the definition of the genetic basis of cystic fibrosis and other genetic disorders is now being employed in the investigation of fragile X syndrome (FMR) and neurofibromatosis (NF). The impact of molecular genetics on our understanding of developmental disabilities and early intervention has the potential to improve significantly the accuracy of diagnosis and the effectiveness of management and counseling.

A key discovery in the field of molecular genetics was bacterial *enzymes* (protein catalysts) called restriction enzymes. These enzymes cut DNA chains into specific fragments, which allows the more precise analysis of DNA.[3,5] This has permitted large chromosomal DNA to be understood as small units of DNA. *Genes* can now be examined and manipulated in units of nucleic acids called nucleotides. This discovery was followed by the development of a number of separation and identification techniques, including *electrophoresis, chromatography,* and *fluorescent staining* to identify fragments of DNA (Fig 1).[3,5] More recent advances have included the development of automated DNA analysis equipment

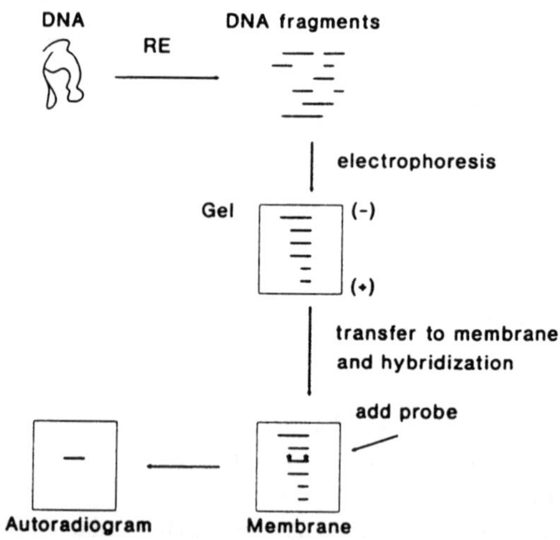

Fig 1. Southern blot analysis. DNA is first digested with a restriction enzyme, and fragments are separated by size and transferred to a membrane. At the hybridization step, the probe binds (**) to the DNA of complementary sequence. After autoradiography, the pattern seen (number of fragments and their size) is characteristic of each enzyme probe combination. Reprinted with permission from: Langlors S. Genetic Diagnosis Based on Molecular Analysis. *Pediatric Clinics of North America.* 1992;39:91–105.

and the technology of *polymerase chain reaction* (PCR), a method to rapidly make multiple choices of an original segment of DNA.[6–8] Before the development of these technologies, analysis of one gene sometimes took years. Today it takes only weeks, and the cost of making DNA copies has dropped precipitously.[9]

In the past, DNA sequencing was hindered by difficulties in obtaining sufficient genetic material for analysis, a process that could take weeks of laborious work.[7] With the development of PCR technology, one piece of DNA (separated from a sample of thousands) can now be duplicated rapidly to make millions of copies within a few hours.[7,8] This technology has made it possible to find a single gene in a drop of blood, a strand of hair, or a plant fiber. New technologies that embed gene-search software programs onto computer chips will speed up the analysis of vast quantities of genetic data.[7]

THE HUMAN GENOME PROJECT

The Human Genome Project was first proposed in the United States by the Department of Education and the National Institutes of Health. Congress established the National Center for Human Genome Research in 1990 with an initial funding of $60 million.[10,11] Scientists met later and established an international organization, the Human Genome Organization, to coordinate human genome research.[4,10–12] Funding for these organizations has come from multiple sources, including the United States Congress, the Hughes Foundation, the Wellcome Foundation, and numerous other governments including those of the United Kingdom, Italy, Japan, and the European community.[3,10]

The overall objective of the Human Genome Project is to map completely the human genome over a 15-year period at a projected cost of $3 billion, or about $200 million dollars per year.[3,4,10] This is equal to about a dollar per *base pair,* or about $30,000 per gene. The more immediate 5-year goals are to obtain a map of human DNA fragments, to assemble DNA sequences, to develop sequencing technology that will reduce cost to $0.25 to $0.50 per base, to develop information technology for database analysis of gene maps and sequencing information, and to formulate comparable technology for sequencing of the genes of other species, such as the mouse.[4,10]

It is estimated that humans have 3×10^9 genes, with 50,000 genes being expressed (known to effect a trait), but only some 5,000 human genes are defined, and only 1,900 have been located on human chromosomes.[2,3] Data on these genes and their *probes* are stored in the genome database maintained in Baltimore at Johns Hopkins University and are available to investigators from the United States, Europe, and Japan via data networks.[2,3] The major databanks are Gen Bank in the United States, EMBL in Europe, and DDBJ in Japan.[2,3,10]

Critics of the Human Genome Project are concerned that a large amount of information is being generated with little specific information about whether it will serve any purpose.[10,13] This is a real concern when basic science funding is shrinking in terms of actual dollars. It is also argued that much information will be obtained about inheritable defects for which no treatment is available and that such information may potentially lead to invasion of privacy and to discrimination in terms of employment and insurance coverage.[10,13]

Proponents of the Human Genome Project argue that the complete map will greatly speed lines of research similar to those that have already led to the identification of genes for cystic fibrosis and muscular dystrophy.[4,5,10–12] It is felt that the rapid identification of human gene loci (locations) will make genetic testing and the prediction of human disease possible even at birth.[10–12] Moreover, the complete gene map may make it easier to define genetic diseases as multifactorial, multigenetic, or nongenetic, which historically has been difficult to determine with real precision.[10–12]

The technology that resulted in the understanding of the genetic basis of cystic fibrosis and muscular dystrophy also has led to the identification of other abnormalities with similar symptoms. Investigators are now beginning to look at potential options for treatment. Investigators in muscular dystrophy research are working on a method to transplant normal muscle cells, called myoblasts, to stabilize the progression of muscle weakness.[13] The use of genetically engineered viruses to carry missing DNA into defective cells lining the surface of the lungs in patients with cystic fibrosis is being explored in an effort to stop the progression of degenerative pulmonary disease.[14]

A committee of the Human Genome Project is also investigating the ethical and legal issues surrounding this research.[10,15] By addressing these concerns, it is felt that the overall program can identify effective policies in a timely manner.[15,16] In addition, the Human Genome Project will encourage the development of technology that will affect the entire field of molecular biology, particularly in the forms of automated equipment and data management.[15,16] It is hoped that worldwide accessibility to a database of genome information will promote cooperation among the medical, biologic, agricultural, and scientific communities and will lead to the interdisciplinary development of necessary hardware and software to manage these large databases.[4,10,16] Many world governments and scientific bodies are presently supporting this project; each of the seven richest nations in the world have committed financial resources and scientific talent.[10]

The technology of molecular genetics is already having an impact on our ability to diagnose inborn disabilities.[5] For example, several genes that cause disorders associated with disabilities recently have been located on specific human chromosomes, such as Huntington's disease on chromosome 4, Werdnig-Hoffmann disease on chromosome 5, spinocerebellar ataxia on chromosome 6, Friedreich's ataxia and tuberous sclerosis on chromosome 9, Wilson's disease on chromosome 13, myotonic dystrophy on chromosome 19, one form of Alzheimer's disease on chromosome 21, and Menkes' syndrome and Lowe syndrome on the X chromosome (Figs 2 and 3). As each month goes by, additional disability-causing genes are being identified on human chromosomes.

Subsequent paragraphs discuss several aspects of molecular genetics that pertain to specific disabilities. These include NF, FMR, phenylketonuria (PKU), the mapping of chromosome 21, and genetic susceptibility and drug metabolism as they relate to fetal drug exposure and birth defects.

NEUROFIBROMATOSIS

NF is a *dominant* disorder, usually appearing in early childhood and affecting multiple organ systems with a wide spectrum of problems.[17,18] Common symptoms include changes in pigmentation (coloration) of the skin and small lumps under the skin called neurofibromas. Complications of NF can be divided into two areas: structural problems such as abnormalities of the bones of the face, head, and spine, and functional disorders including seizures, speech disorders, cognitive deficits, learning disabilities, and high blood pressure.[17,18] Severe complications include malignant and nonmalignant tumors, particularly in the visual system and the brain.

The gene for type 1 neurofibromatosis (NF-1) has been located at a specific region of chromosome 17.[1,19,20] The NF-1 gene extends across about 300,000 bases of DNA and codes for the synthesis of a large protein of about 2,818 amino acids.[19,20] Active research continues in an effort to understand fully this gene and its functions. It is felt that this information will be useful in the diagnosis of both inherited (familial) and sporadic cases of NF-1. DNA testing for *prenatal markers* in children at risk of inheriting NF-1 and for diagnosis of individuals who have mild cases of NF is currently possible. As research continues on the NF-1 protein synthesized by this gene, we may begin to understand more about its role in the functions of the central nervous system.

FRAGILE X SYNDROME

FMR, originally called sex-linked mental retardation, appears as moderate to profound mental retardation in many males and as borderline to mild mental retardation in some females.[17,18,21] The gene that leads to FMR (FMR-1) is a major cause of mental retardation and has been mapped to the X chromosome.[1,5,21,22] The sequencing of the FMR-1 gene has identified an unstable repeating sequence of the *nucleic acids* within a region of that gene (in this case, base pairs of cytosine and guanine in a CGG sequence; see *A,T,C,G* in the glossary).[23] Research has revealed that the region on the chromosome that contains the FMR-1 gene grows from generation to generation.[24] As the number of repetitive sequences of CGG increases, the severity of the disorder also increases.[25] *Carriers* have a smaller

Chromosome 3

von Hippel-Lindau syndrome

Chromosome 4

Huntington's disease

Facioscapulohumeral muscular dystrophy

Chromosome 5

Werdnig-Hoffmann disease

Familial polyposis coli*

Chromosome 6

Spinocerebellar ataxia-1

Chromosome 7

Cystic fibrosis*

Chromosome 9

Friedreich's ataxia

Tuberous sclerosis-1

Chromosome 10

Multiple endocrine neoplasia II

Chromosome 11

Beckwith-Wiedemann syndrome

Wilms' tumor*

Aniridia-2

Multiple endocrine neoplasia I

Ataxia-telangiectasia

Chromosome 13

Retinoblastoma*

Wilson's disease

Chromosome 15

Marfan syndrome*

Chromosome 16

Polycystic kidney disease

*Gene cloned

Chromosome 17

Miller-Dieker lissencephaly syndrome

Charcot-Marie-Tooth disease-1a

von Recklinghausen neurofibromatosis*

Early-onset breast cancer

Chromosome 19

Myotonic dystrophy

Chromosome 20

Maturity-onset diabetes of the young

Chromosome 21

Amyotrophic lateral sclerosis (one form)

Alzheimer's disease (one form)

Chromosome 22

Acoustic neuroma (NF2)

X Chromosome

Kallmann syndrome

Retinoschisis

Chronic granulomatous disease*

Duchenne type muscular dystrophy*

Norrie's disease

Incontinentia pigmenti

Wiskott-Aldrich syndrome

Menkes' syndrome

Agammaglobulinemia

Choroideremia

Alport-like hereditary nephritis

Lowe syndrome

Fragile X syndrome*

Adrenoleukodystrophy

Emery-Dreifuss muscular dystrophy

Y Chromosome

XY gonadal dysgenesis*

Fig 2. Recent and current targets of positional cloning in the human genome. Reprinted with permission from: Collins F.S. Identification of Disease Genes: Recent Success. *Hospital Practice.* 1991;26:93–98.

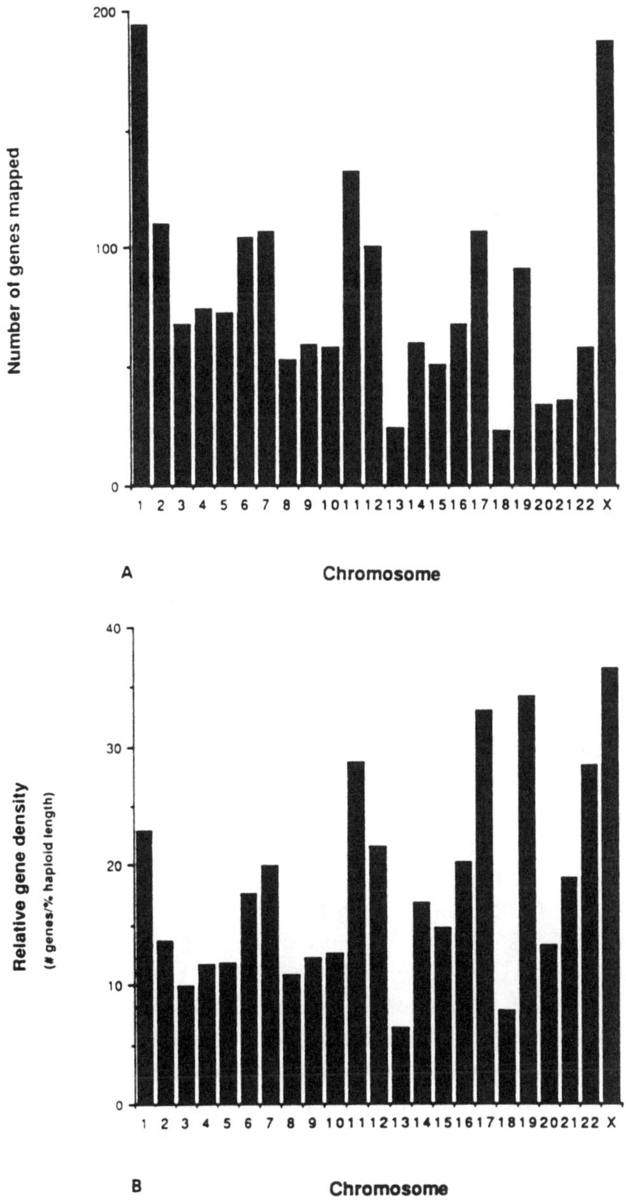

Fig 3. (**A**) Number of gene assignments by chromosome. (**B**) Relative density of genes assigned to each chromosome. Reprinted with permission from: McKusick V.A. Current Trends in Mapping Human Genes. *The FASEB Journal.* 1991;5:12–20.

number of repetitive sequences, but individuals with the disorder have more than 200 and sometimes up to 1,000 repetitive CGG sequences. With an increasing number of repetitions of the CGG sequence, there is a decreasing production of the FMR-1 protein.[25] The specific function of the FMR-1 protein is not known; but the absence of this protein is related to the features of FMR.[21,25]

The identification of the FMR-1 region has led to the development of DNA probes (small pieces of DNA of known sequence) that, coupled with PCR technology, has resulted in accurate identification of affected and carrier males and females.[24,25] This DNA testing can identify many more carriers than were previously recognized.[21,24] The use of these DNA probes has also allowed the tracking of mutations through a number of generations.[21,24] DNA testing in individuals with mental retardation and autism of unknown cause could be extremely helpful in early identification of the genetic basis for developmental delay.[21,25] This type of genetic analysis is also appropriate in families with affected members to allow prenatal counseling.[17,24,25]

DOWN SYNDROME AND MAPPING OF CHROMOSOME 21

Down syndrome, a major cause of mental retardation, is caused by an excess of chromosome 21 material.[17,18] Children with Down syndrome may have various disorders, including developmental delay, low muscle tone, and disorders of the skin, eyes, gastrointestinal system, endocrine system, and heart. Major anomalies of the gastrointestinal tract and heart and recurrent respiratory infections are major causes of illness and death.[17,26]

A number of research techniques have been used to investigate the molecular basis of Down syndrome and to map chromosome 21.[27–31] Recently, efforts have focused on the genes responsible for the physical disorders associated with Down syndrome, such as congenital heart disease and an intestinal blockage called duodenal atresia.[30] Genetic maps show that specific regions of chromosome 21 form the molecular basis for the physical symptoms of Down syndrome[28–31] Mapping of chromosome 21 and defining the correlations between specific genes and physical traits in Down syndrome are presently underway.[27]

DNA probes have recently been used to determine the parental origin of extra chromosomal material and other associated chromosomal errors. DNA probe analysis has shown that extra chromosomal material in Down syndrome is maternal in origin in 94% of cases and paternal in the remaining 6%.[32] These data are considered more accurate than earlier cytogenetic data. The use of molecular probes has also shown that in nearly 75% of the cases the maternal chromosomal error occurs in the first meiotic (reduction) division of gametes (eggs) in the mother's fetal life.[33] In the other 25%, the chromosomal error occurs in adult life, at the time of the second meiotic division during ovulation. There appears to be no correlation between the mother's age at the time of conception and the stage of meiosis during which the error occurs.[33]

PHENYLKETONURIA

PKU was one of the first metabolic disorders to be defined, and in the search for an intervention it served as a prime motivator for the development of *metabolic screening* programs for newborns.[5] PKU is a *recessive* disorder caused by a deficiency of the liver enzyme phenylalanine hydroxylase (PAH).[5,34] The disorder is characterized by excess phenylalanine, the accumulation of phenylalanine in tissues, and abnormalities in amino acid metabolism. Individuals with untreated PKU develop irreversible mental retardation. The frequency of PKU ranges from 1:10,000 in the white population to 1:120,000 in the Japanese population; about 1 person in 50 carries this gene.[34,35]

By means of molecular techniques, 60 specific mutations of the PAH gene have been determined.[34] Of these, 95% cannot be detected by present metabolic screening methods.[34,36–38] of these 60 mutations, 50 involve a mutation in a single base pair.[34] Present mapping techniques have located the gene for PAH on chromosome 12.[1,34,38] Molecular analysis has shown that the PAH gene is a 90,000-base piece of DNA.[34] Analyses of common mutations of the PAH gene show a significant correlation between the amount of PAH activity and the symptoms of the disease. A clear relationship exists between the symptoms of PKU, PAH levels in the blood, and protein tolerance after eating high-protein foods.[34,38] Molecular genetic techniques have been remarkably successful in identifying and understanding the mutations of the PAH gene.

Of even greater interest are the prospects for the application of these techniques to the characterization of the *promoter region* that regulates the activities of the human PAH gene. Abnormalities in this particular region may explain other PAH deficiencies and may provide information useful for the detection of other mutations in patients with PKU.[34] The identification of these mutations is important not only for identifying regions that regulate PAH gene expression but also for understanding the molecular basis of PKU, related disorders, and developmental concerns associated with excess phenylalanine.

These molecular techniques are useful not only in defining the role of PKU and PAH in the developing nervous system but also in improving our understanding of other metabolic disorders that involve mental retardation. In the future, it is likely that molecular techniques will evolve into diagnostic tests that will either augment or replace traditional metabolic screening as the best way to detect and track mutations in families with these disorders.

GENETIC SUSCEPTIBILITY TO THE EFFECTS OF FETAL DRUG EXPOSURE

Many children with birth defects also have major abnormalities of the developing central nervous system that result in significant developmental, cognitive, and learning problems. Birth defects caused by drug exposure or other toxins have been described only in the last 15 years.[39–41] Research has documented that individuals are affected in different ways by drug exposure before birth. For some fetuses this can translate into congenital birth defects.[42–44] Initial studies in the molecular genetics of *biotransformation* and *pharmacogenetics* suggest that fetal drug exposure may disrupt several major enzyme systems.[42–47] These enzyme systems are generalized in their activity and could be affected not only by anticonvulsant medications but also by other drugs and toxins.

Phenytoin is a major anticonvulsant that has been used to treat epilepsy for more than 50 years. It has been used extensively in the treatment of pregnant women. The adverse effects of phenytoin on fetal *morphogenesis* (organ development) have been reported by a number of investigators.[39,48] Clinical studies of fetal phenytoin syndrome have shown that fetal susceptibility to phenytoin exposure is highly variable.[41] In humans, phenytoin is metabolized from chemical substances that may affect fetal development; then it is oxidized to form products for excretion.[42]

Molecular genetics techniques are used to study major enzyme systems and to establish point mutations (single base changes) that may result in genetic susceptibility to fetal drug exposure.[48,49] Although point mutations may be frequent in the general population and may not result in problems in the individual taking the medication, they may play a role in the metabolizing of a medication into chemicals that are toxic to the fetus, resulting in birth defects.[38] Molecular genetics will be invaluable in providing greater insight into the effects of exposure to medications and other toxins on the fetus during pregnancy. These techniques may, in addition, provide prenatal markers to identify women at risk.[42]

• • •

Advances in molecular genetics will continue to have an impact on the diagnosis and understanding of a number of developmental disorders. In the future, this technology may provide greater insight into specific problems such as susceptibility to fetal drug exposure and congenital malformations and may aid in both preventing and treating disabilities. Although this article has covered only a few developmental disabilities, the techniques of molecular genetics described here are being applied to a long list of conditions. Molecular genetics is broadening our understanding of specific diseases and conditions. It has taken us from understanding how we inherit hair and eye color, to recognizing specific patterns of malformation, to identifying alterations in the genetic code that lead to defects in the body's basic biochemistry and organ system development.

Our present understanding has opened new avenues of exploration for possible treatment and prevention. At the present time, treatments are restricted to the areas of bone marrow transplantation, myoblast transfer, and the experimental use of genetically engineered adenoviruses to incorporate DNA into defective cells. Information provided through the Human Genome Project and other projects in clinical and basic science are expanding our ability to diagnose, manage, treat, and prevent developmental disabilities.

REFERENCES

1. Collins FS. Identification of disease genes: recent success. *Hosp Pract.* 1991;26:93–98.
2. McKusick VA. Current trends in mapping human genes. *FASEB J.* 1991;5:12–20.
3. McKusick VA. Genomic mapping and how it has progressed. *Hosp Pract.* 1991;26;74–90.
4. Watson JD. The Human Genome Project: past, present, and future. *Science.* 1990;248:44–49.
5. Langlors S. Genetic diagnosis based on molecular analysis. *Pediatr Clin North Am.* 1992;39:91–105.
6. Rossiter BJF, Caskey CT. Molecular studies of human genetic disease. *FASEB J.* 1991;5:21–27.
7. Rose EA. Applications of the polymerase chain reaction to genome analysis. *FASEB J.* 1991;5:46–54.
8. Billings PR, Smith CL, Canter CR. New techniques for physical mapping of the human genome. *FASEB J.* 1991;5:28–34.
9. Gilbert W. DNA sequencing, today and tomorrow. *Hosp Pract.* 1991;26:165–174.
10. Flannagan JR. The Human Genome Project (HGP): implications for medicine and the public. Presented at a clinical epidemiological symposium: Assuring Quality Medical Care: Toward the Year 2000; October 31, 1991; University of Iowa, Iowa City.
11. Watson JD. ASHG Human Genome Committee Report, The Human Genome Project: implications for human genetics. *Am J Hum Genet.* 1991;49:687–691.
12. Stephens JC, Cavanaugh ML, Gradie MI, Mador ML, Kidd KK. Mapping the human genome: current status. *Science.* 1990;250:237–244.
13. Law PK, Goodwin TG, Fang Q, et al. Feasibility, safety, and efficacy of myoblast transfer therapy on Duchenne muscular dystrophy boys. *Cell Transform.* 1992;1:235–244.
14. Rosenfeld MA, Crystal RG, Trapnell BC, et al. In vivo transfer of the human cystic fibrosis transmembrane conductance regulator gene to the airway epithelium. *Cell.* 1992;68:143–155.
15. Wexler NS. Disease gene identification: ethical considerations. *Hosp Pract.* 1991;26:145–152.
16. Watson JD. The human genome initiative: a statement of need. *Hosp Pract.* 1991;26:69–73.
17. Jones KL. *Smith's Recognizable Patterns of Human Malformation* (4th ed). Philadelphia, Pa: Saunders; 1988.
18. Goodman RM, Gorlin RJ. *The Malformed Infant and Child: An Illustrated Guide.* New York, NY: Oxford University Press; 1983.

19. Cawthon RM, Weiss R, Xu G, et al. A major segment of the neurofibromatosis type 1 gene: DNA sequence, genome structure and point mutations. *Cell.* 1990;62:193–201.

20. Wallace MR, Marchuk DA, Anderson LB, et al. Type 1 neurofibromatosis gene: identification of a large transcript description in three NF1 patients. *Science.* 1990;249:181–186.

21. Goldson E, Hagerman RJ. The fragile X syndrome. *Dev Med Child Neurol.* 1992;34:822–832.

22. Turner G, Daniel A, Frost M. X-Linked mental retardation, macroorchidism and the Xq27 fragile site. *J Pediatr.* 1989;96:837–841.

23. Snow K, Dond L, Hagerman R, et al. Analysis of mutation of the fragile X locus using the DNA probe OX19. *Am J Med Genet.* 1992;43:244–254.

24. Verkerk AJMH, Pieretti M. Sutcliffe JS, et al. Identification of a gene (FMR-1) containing a CGG repeat coincidental with a breakpoint cluster region exhibiting length variation in fragile X syndrome. *Cell.* 1991;65:905–914.

25. Rousseau F, Heitz D, Biancaloni V, et al. Direct diagnosis by DNA analysis of the fragile X syndrome of mental retardation. *N Engl J Med.* 1991;325:1673–1681.

26. Antonarakis SE. Down Syndrome Collaborative Group, parental origin of the extra chromosome in trisomy 21 as indicated by analysis of DNA polymorphisms. *N Engl J Med.* 1991;324:872–876.

27. Tanzi RE, Watkins PC, Stewart CG, Wexler NS, Gusella JF, Haines JL. A genetic linkage map of human chromosome 21: analysis of recombination as a function of sex and age. *Am J Hum Genet.* 1992;50:551–558.

28. Epstein CJ, Korenberg JR, Anneren G, et al. Protocols to establish genotype-phenotype correlations in Down syndrome. *Am J Human Genet.* 1991;49:207–235.

29. Korenberg JR, Kawashima H, Pulst SM, et al. Molecular definition of a region of chromosome 21 that causes features of the Down syndrome phenotype. *Am J Hum Genet.* 1990;47:236–246.

30. Korenberg JR, Bradley C, Disteche CM. Down syndrome: molecular mapping of congenital heart disease and duodenal stenosis. *Am J Hum Genet.* 1992;50:294–302.

31. Korenberg JR, Kawashima H, Pulst SM, Allen L, Magenis E, Epstein CJ. Down syndrome: toward a molecular definition of the phenotype. *Am J Med Genet.* 1990;7(suppl):91–97.

32. Sherman SL, Takaesu N, Freeman SB, et al. Trisomy 21: association between reduced recombination and nondisjunction. *Am J Hum Genet.* 1991;49:608–620.

33. Antonarakis SE, Petersen MB, McInnis MG, et al. The meiotic stage of nondisjunction in trisomy 21: determination by using DNA polymorphisms. *Am J Hum Genet.* 1992;50:544–550.

34. Eisensmith RG, Woo SLC. Molecular basis of phenylketonuria and related hyperphenylalaninemia; mutations and polymorphisms in the human phenylalanine hydroxylase gene. *Hum Mutat.* 1992;1:13–23.

35. Konecki DS, Lichter-Konecki U. The phenylketonuria locus: current knowledge about alleles and mutations of the phenylalanine hydroxylase gene in various populations. *Hum Genet.* 1991;87:389–393.

36. Lidsky AS, Law ML, Morse HG, Kao FT, Woo SLC. Regional mapping of the phenylalanine hydroxylase gene and the phenylketonuria locus in the human genome. *Proc Natl Acad Sci USA.* 1985;82:6221–6225.

37. Dwornicak B, Aulehla-Scholz C, Horst J. Phenylalanine hydroxylase gene: silent mutation uncovers evolutionary origin of different alleles. *Clin Genet.* 1990;38:270–273.

38. Okano Y, Eisensmith RC, Guttler F, et al. Molecular basis of phenotype heterogenicity in PKU. *N Engl J Med.* 1991;324:1232–1238.

39. Kelly TE. Teratogenicity of anticonvulsant drugs—review of the literature. *Am J Med Genet.* 1987;19:413–434.

40. Hanson J. Teratogen update: fetal hydantoin effects. *Teratology.* 1986;33:349–353.

41. Van Dyke DC, Hodge SR, Heide F, Hill LR. Family studies in fetal phenytoin exposure. *J Pediatr.* 1988;113:301–306.

42. Van Dyke DC, Berg MJ, Olson CH. Differences in phenytoin biotransformation and susceptibility to congenital malformations: a review. *Ann Pharmacother.* 1991;25:987–992.

43. Spielberg SP, Gordon GB, Blake DA, Goldstein DA, Herlong F. Predisposition of phenytoin hepatoxicity addressed in vitro. *N Engl J Med.* 1981;305:722–727.

44. Stickler SM, Miller MA, Anderson E, Danaky LV, Sem MH, Spielberg SP. Genetic predisposition to phenytoin-induced birth defects. *Lancet.* 1985;2:746–799.

45. Skoda RC, Demierre A, McBride OW, Gonzales FJ, Meyer UA. Human microsomal xenobiotic epoxide hydrolase. *J Biol Chem.* 1988;263:1549–1557.

46. Gonzales FJ, Newbert DW. Evolution of the P450 gene super family: animal-plant "warfare," molecular drive and human genetic differences in drug oxidation. *Trends Genet.* 1990;6:182–186.

47. Buehler BA, Delimont D, Van Wess M, Finnell RH. Prenatal prediction of risk of the fetal hydantoin syndrome. *N Engl J Med.* 1990;322:1567–1572.

48. Gough AC, Miles JS, Spurr NK, et al. Identification of the primary gene defect at the cytochrome P450 CYP2D locus. *Nature (London).* 1990;347:773–776.

49. Hanioka N, Shioko K, Meyer VA, Gonzales FJ. The human CYP2D locus associated with a common gene defect in drug oxidation: a G1934-A base change intron 3 of a mutant CYP2D6 allele results in an aberrant 3' A splice recognition site. *Am J Hum Genet.* 1990;47:994–1001.

Appendix
Glossary

A,T,C,G—The basic building blocks of DNA. A, adenine; T, thymine; C, cystine; G, guanine.

Amino Acids—Chemical compounds that are the structural units of proteins. Proteins are important building blocks of cells, which make up our bodies. There are many different types of amino acids units. Those amino acids that have a large ring structure are called aromatic amino acids. Phenylalanine is an aromatic amino acid.

Base Pair or Bases—The complementary bonding of nucleotides. The bases of DNA are adenine, thymine, cytosine, and guanine. Because DNA is a three-dimensional structure, DNA molecules pair with a partner. For example, adenine bonds with its complementary partner thymine, and cytosine bonds with its complementary partner guanine. Base pairing allows DNA to have the three-dimensional structure needed to carry large amounts of genetic information and for replication.

Biotransformation—The process whereby bacteria, plant, or animal cells biochemically alter the structure of a chemical compound.

Carrier—A person who carries the genes for a trait and who can pass on these genes but who does not have the symptoms or physical characteristics associated with that trait. Some genes are dominant, which means that they are always expressed, and some genes are recessive, which means that they are expressed when there are two doses of the gene. In a carrier state, a person carries a normal gene and an abnormal gene. The abnormal gene is not expressed but is detectable by a laboratory test.

Chromatography—A technique for separating chemical compounds based on their migration through a medium such as agar, gelatin, or paper, and their relative solubility in a specific solvent such as water or alcohol. Variations in solubility and size allow many compounds to be separated by this technique.

Chromosomes—Structures within the nucleus of a cell that are made up of proteins (primarily histones) and DNA. When one looks under the microscope, chromosomes present as definable structures with a center and two arms. The smaller arm is abbreviated p; the longer arm is abbreviated q. The arms are divided into small segments based on staining properties called bands, which are usually expressed as a number (eg, q22).

Cytogenetics—The study of the microscopic appearance of chromosomes, their function, and their replication.

DNA—Deoxyribonucleic acid, the memory bank for all cells. DNA resembles a protein in that it is constructed from building blocks. These building blocks contain a phosphate group, a sugar (deoxyribose), and a base (adenine, guanine, cytosine, or thymine). DNA has a three-dimensional configuration that allows information to be copied precisely and passed on from cell to cell.

Electrophoresis—The technique of separating chemical compounds such as DNA or proteins in electrical fields based on their differences in charge.

Enzyme—Proteins that catalyze biochemical reactions.

Expression—Genes code for specific factors, specifically proteins, which may have specific functions. The presence or absence of genetic information, whether the end result is eye color, hair color, skin color or lack of skin color, or eye or hair color, is called expression.

Fluorescent Staining—Fluorescence is a property whereby dyes, when exposed to various wavelengths of light, glow (fluorescence). The ability of certain compounds to take up fluorescent stains allows them to be identified when exposed to various wavelengths of light.

Gene—A gene is composed of highly specific segments of DNA. There are structural genes and regulatory genes. In structural genes, nucleotides code for a specific coding unit. Each unit is translated into a specific amino acid. Proteins are made up of amino acids. Proteins are those chemical compounds that make up the structure of cells.

Genotype—Specific genetic information that an individual carries (genetic constitution or genome).

Human Genome Project—Started in 1990 with a goal of determining and locating specific pieces of DNA on chromosomes. The term *genome* refers to small pieces of genetic information (genes) that are located on the chromosomes. In short, the project's major goal is to determine the structure of different genes, what they code for, and where they are located on the chromosome.

Metabolic Screening—A number of inborn errors in metabolism have been identified. The method for identifying them is called metabolic screening. Metabolic screening consists of a number of techniques and tests for identification of abnormalities of metabolism. In most states, newborns are screened in the first 2 or 3 days of life for inborn errors of metabolism.

Morphogenesis—The evolution and development of forms as cells develop into organs.

Mutation—Permanent heritable changes in DNA. Point mutations are single base mutations.

Nucleotide—The building blocks of nucleic acids. They contain a phosphate group, a sugar and a base (adenine, thymine, cytosine, or guanine).

Pharmacogenetics—The study of alterations of DNA (mutations) that may lead to changes in metabolism of drugs (medications).

Phenotype—The entire physical, physiologic, and biochemical make-up of an individual as determined by genetic constitution and environmental influences.

Polymerase Chain Reaction (PCR)—A technique that uses a special bacterial enzyme called a polymerase to make millionfold copies of a piece of DNA. The process of making multiple copies of a specific DNA fragment is called amplification.

Prenatal Markers—Segments of DNA. Certain markers are inherited with certain diseases. They can be used prenatally in some cases to help determine the inheritance of certain diseases.

Probes—Known sequences of (usually small) pieces of DNA.

Promoter Region—In addition to structural genes, we have what are called regulatory genes. One specific type of regulator is called a promoter. Specifically, promoters are the start signals for RNA synthesis.

Sequencing—Determining the order of bases in DNA or of amino acids in a protein.

Toxicology—The study of poisons, their action, their detection, and the treatment of conditions produced by them.

Topographic brain mapping: A window on brain function?

Walt M. Karniski, MD
Associate Professor and Director
Section of Child Development
Department of Pediatrics
University of South Florida College of Medicine
Tampa, Florida

A LARGE NUMBER of disorders of the central nervous system (CNS) significantly impair human behavior without affecting the normal macrostructure of the brain. Although technologic accomplishments have produced accurate, noninvasive representations of three-dimensional brain structure (computed tomography [CT], magnetic resonance imaging [MRI], sonogram), these techniques have been of limited value in the clinical assessment of disorders of CNS function.

This has been particularly evident in infants and children. Most studies of childhood developmental disorders (eg, cerebral palsy, autism, learning disorders, dyslexia, childhood schizophrenia) have revealed no evidence of consistent structural abnormalities that would assist the clinician in differential diagnosis.

However, a new technique, topographic mapping of quantitative EEG, or brain mapping, may be a physiologic window on brain function. Brain mapping may have great potential for better understanding and differentiation of developmental disorders in children. This article will explain the basic principles behind topographic brain mapping and will attempt to explore the potential application to infants and children.

FREQUENCY MAPPING

For any measure that changes systematically in space, a map can be created. For instance, the colored weather maps that appear daily in newspapers document the temperature changes in different parts of the country. In the same way topographic brain maps produce visual representations of the changes in electrical activity across the human scalp.

The standard EEG is produced by measuring the voltage differences between electrodes at many sites across the surface of the scalp and some reference electrode. The waveforms produced by an EEG indicate voltage changes over time (frequency) and over the scalp (topography). Topographic brain mapping attempts to condense the information produced by a traditional EEG on pages of waveform tracings into maps that can be more readily assimilated.

The author acknowledges Loretta Lease, R EEGT, and Lucia Grimaldi, BA who assisted in the preparation of this article.

Inf Young Children 1989; 1(3): 63–76

Frequency maps

Most of the activity in the frequency spectrum of the EEG occurs between 0 and 25 cycles per second (Hz). Traditionally the frequency spectrum has been divided into four main subgroups (Fig 1): delta (0.5 to 3.5 Hz), theta (4.0 to 7.5 Hz), alpha (8.0 to 13.0 Hz), and beta (13.5 to 25.0 Hz). These subgroupings have been found to have functional significance. For instance, if an individual is relaxed and alert,

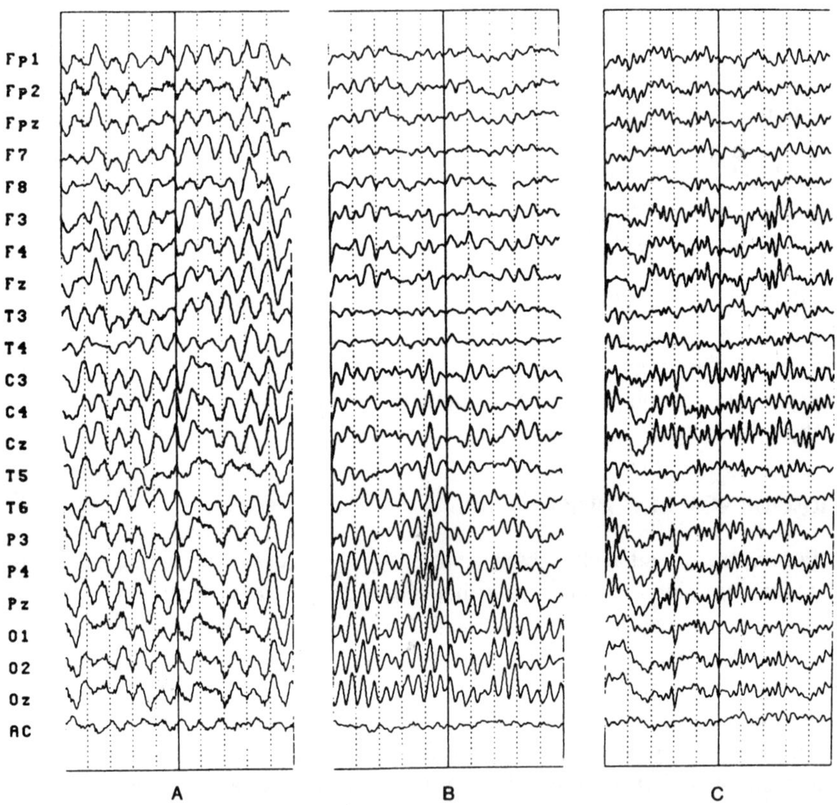

Fig 1. Traditional EEG. Three samples of EEG activity demonstrate the complex frequencies making up a typical EEG. Five- to six-cycle-per-second theta activity is seen in the first trace (**A**). The second example (**B**) reveals very rhythmic, high-voltage alpha in the posterior region, with slower, lower voltage activity more anterior. The last example reveals much faster, lower-voltage beta activity (**C**). However, the waves are complex, overlapping, and constantly changing. All traces were from the same subject using 21 electrodes referenced to linked-ear electrodes. (See **Fig 4A** for electrode placements.)

with eyes closed, the dominant frequency will be alpha, seen primarily in the posterior occipital region. If the eyes are then opened, occipital alpha disappears and is replaced by faster beta activity. During sleep the background frequencies take on characteristic appearances, then slow with increasing amounts of theta activity as the individual slips into deeper stages of sleep. Dreaming occurs during rapid eye movement (REM) sleep, and the background rhythms are more consistent with the activity seen in the awake EEG. An injured brain can produce many different types of EEG findings, but an increase in delta in the area of the injury is often seen.

However, the EEG signal is rarely a simple sine wave with regular peaks and valleys, so that characterization of the frequency of the EEG is not easy. More often there are multiple frequencies with different voltages simultaneously superimposed. A simplified example is shown in Fig 2. A sine wave with a frequency of 10 Hz (Fig 2A) has been added to another sine wave with one third the amplitude and a frequency of 2 Hz (Fig 2B) to produce a more complex wave (Fig 2C).

Any wave, no matter how complex, can be mathematically approximated by the sum of a finite number of sine or cosine waves of different amplitude.[1] Computer-

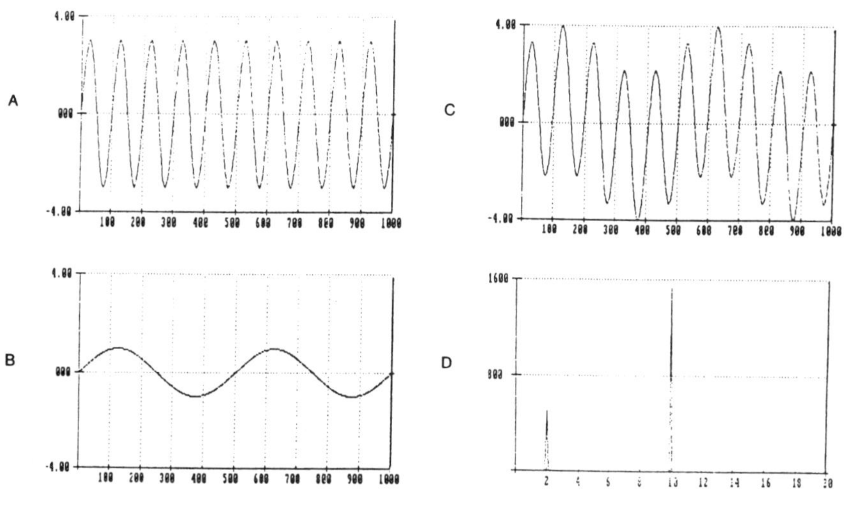

Fig 2. Frequency analysis for simple waves. Any wave, no matter how complex, can be mathematically broken down into sine and cosine wave components. A simple example is illustrated. A sine wave with frequency of 10 Hz (**A**) is added to a sine wave with frequency of 2 Hz (**B**) with amplitude equal to one third of that in (A) to produce a more complex wave (**C**; time in milliseconds on the X-axis, voltage in microvolts on the Y-axis). A frequency *v* power (microvolts squared) plot (**D**) indicates two "pure" peaks, one at 10 Hz and a second at 2 Hz. Power measurements reflect relative amplitude differences of initial waves.

ized quantitative EEG analysis takes advantage of a technique called the fast Fourier transform, or FFT, to break waveforms down into their frequency components. The result of an FFT analysis plots frequency on the X-axis and power on the Y-axis. The power is a measure of the quantity of a given frequency produced by the sine and cosine-squared sums and is expressed in terms of voltage squared. In Fig 2, wave 2C has been analyzed by FFT, producing a power spectrum plot (Fig 2D). Two peaks are seen, a small peak at 2 Hz and a larger one at 10 Hz proportionate to the amplitude difference of the original waves. Through this method any waveform can be broken down into its frequency components. An actual EEG wave can be seen to be much more complex (Fig 3). In this case predominant alpha activity (8 to 12 Hz) is overlapped by faster, low-voltage fast beta activity (which is often an artifact produced by muscle activity) and a slow undulation of the wave at approximately 3 Hz.

To generate a topographic map of EEG power, multiple electrodes across the scalp are used. Numerous segments of spontaneous EEG are chosen, with specific care taken to avoid segments with nonneural artifacts, such as the slow waves produced frontally from eye movement or the rapid waves generated by muscle movement. FFTs are performed on each segment, then averaged together to produce a frequency-power graph for each electrode (eg, Fig 3B). Then a single power value for each preset frequency band (beta, alpha, theta, and delta) is generated by measuring the area under the curve between the limits of the frequency band. For different clinical and experimental applications, the frequency bands can be established with different limits, or more frequent divisions with smaller bands can be employed. For example, the background rhythm of infants and children is much slower than adults with the average dominant posterior rhythm of a 6-month-old in the range of four to five Hz. Thus smaller, lower frequency bands would be more desirable when studying children.

These techniques reduce the large amount of data into a set of four single numbers for each electrode. Now four different topographic maps can be generated, one for each frequency band. In Fig 4A the electrode locations on a schematic of the head are displayed. In Fig 4B they are replaced with their respective power values at each point, as determined by FFT analysis, and isopower lines are then drawn in from a series of linear interpolations to delineate the contours (Fig 4B). In the final step, a color or, for this article, increasing shades of gray are assigned to graded levels of power. The result is a color or gray-scale topographic map (Fig 4C). It is important to emphasize that the topographic map still contains the same information initially available, but now it is presented in such a way that the topographic relationships are more easily assimilated.

The same process is carried out for each of the specified frequency bands, and the result is four maps summarizing the absolute power relationships across the head for each band (Fig 5A). Relative power maps display the relative contribu-

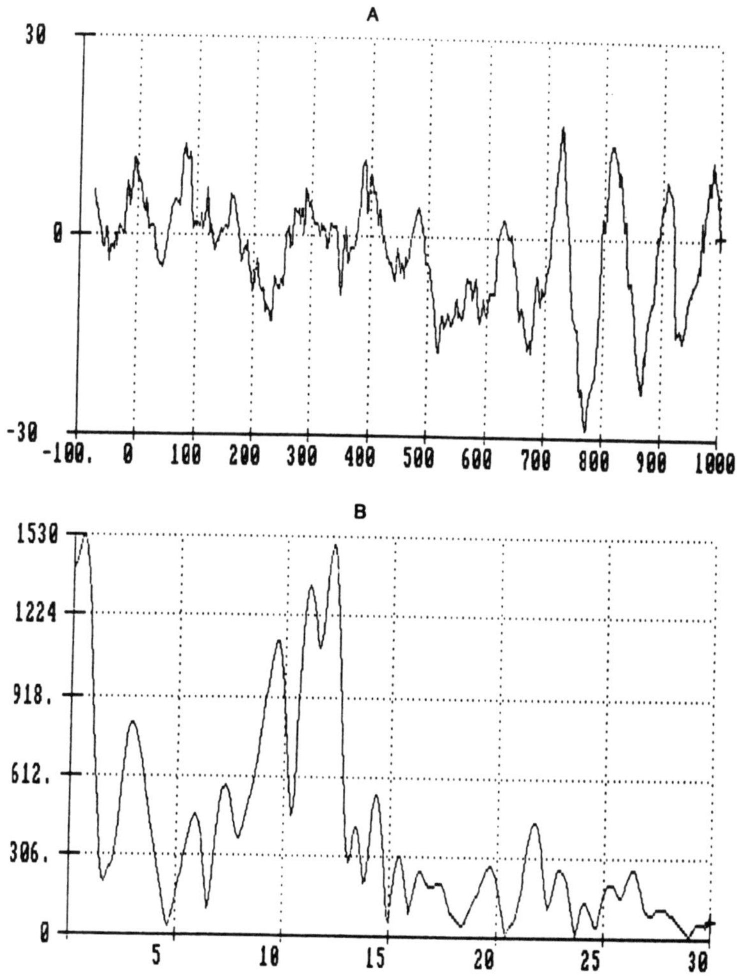

Fig 3. Frequency analysis for complex waves. A raw EEG sample (**A**) is subjected to fast Fourier transform to produce an FFT spectrum plot (**B**), indicating the more complex breakdown of waveform frequency. If the waveform is inspected visually, 11 or 12 prominent peaks can be counted, and this is confirmed by the FFT plot, which indicates that most of the spectral activity is in the alpha range, here 8 to 12 Hz. However, the waves are not smooth, and low-voltage faster activity is superimposed on the slower alpha waves at 20 to 28 Hz, probably a combination of beta and muscle activity. Finally, a slow weaving of the wave at the rate of 2 to 3 cycles per second is reflected in the 3-Hz peak in the spectral plot (**A:** time in milliseconds on the X-axis, voltage in microvolts on the Y-axis; **B:** frequency in hertz on the X-axis, power in microvolts squared on the Y-axis).

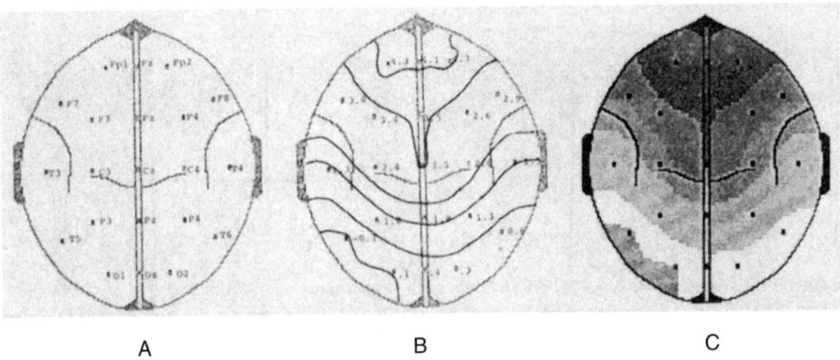

Fig 4. Topographic mapping. The electrode locations are laid out upon a schematic representation of the scalp (**A**). Power values are placed at each electrode site, and isopower lines are added to produce a contour map (**B**). Divisions created by the isopower lines are assigned colors or various shades of gray along a spectrum to represent the power at each point on the map (**C**). (Anterior up, left hemisphere is on the left.)

tions of each band to the total power by dividing the power at each electrode by the total power (or total area under the curve) in all bands at each electrode (Fig 5B). Asymmetries in power between hemispheres can be visualized by an asymmetry index generated by subtracting the power at one electrode on the right from the homologous electrode on the left and dividing by the sum of the two (Fig 5C). The asymmetry maps will always be mirror images of each other because if the power at the left electrode is greater than the right, the power at the right electrode is obviously less than the left by an equal amount.

Once these numerous maps have been created and studied for any length of time, the most obvious question is "What is the expected appearance of the topographic maps for the average person without evidence of neurologic dysfunction?" When a radiologist examines a skull radiograph, there are certain findings that are clearly abnormal, some that are clearly normal, and others that occur inconsistently, and that under certain conditions are considered normal findings. However, the radiologist is looking for structural abnormalities and is often able to obtain confirmation over time through surgery or autopsy findings. Such feedback may not be available for maps of functional CNS activity. In lieu of that database of information, built up over years of clinical practice, statistical analysis of neurologically normal, asymptomatic individuals has been used to establish a normal database.[2-4] This is even more crucial in the pediatric population because even a few years will mean dramatic changes in EEG frequency and topography.[5]

A Z score is a measure of a single subject's frequency deviation from the mean of a comparison population in terms of number of standard deviations.

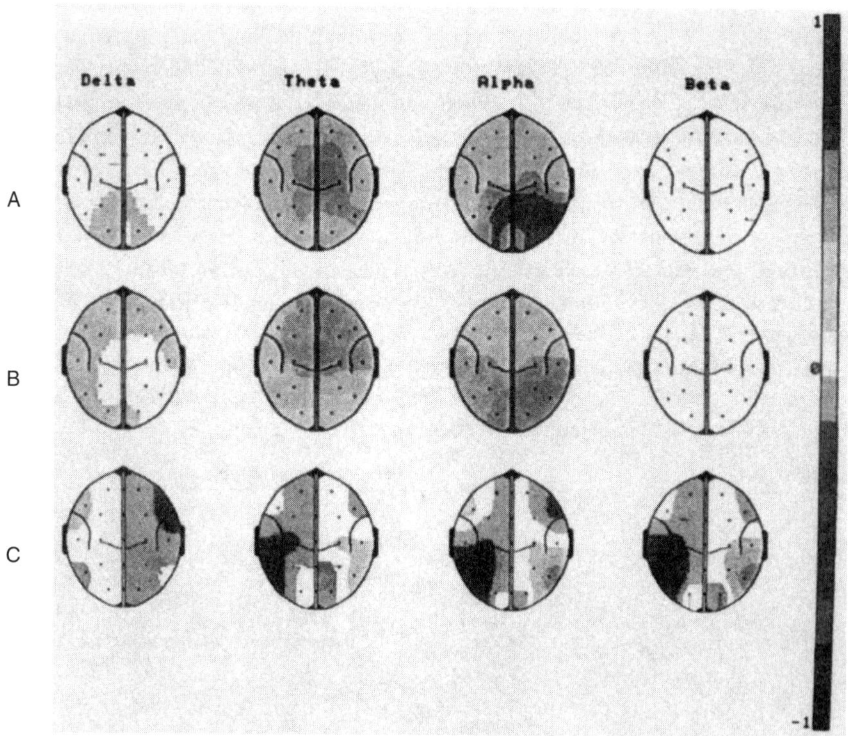

Fig 5. Quantitative EEG analysis for one subject. The four frequency bands are displayed in the columns. The first row is absolute power in microvolts (**A**). The second row is of relative power maps (**B;** power in each frequency band divided by total power across all frequency bands). The last row shows asymmetry maps (**C**), produced by taking the difference between homologous electrodes divided by the sum of the two.

$$Z = \frac{P - \overline{P}}{SD}$$

where P = the power of the subject at one electrode, $\overline{P}$ = the mean power of a comparison population at that electrode, and SD = the standard deviation of the comparison population's power at that point. Thus a Z score of 2.3 indicates that the subject's value is 2.3 SDs above the mean, while a Z score of –1.7 would indicate a value 1.7 SDs below the mean. The maps in Fig 5 have more meaning if they are converted into Z maps[4] (Fig 6). Values between 2 and –2 are left blank, whereas the areas outside of those boundaries are proportionately shaded.

A clinical case study

It is important to understand that a statistical increase or decrease of power from certain electrodes does not necessarily imply that an abnormality of brain function underlies those electrodes. Few controlled studies have validated this technique in clinical populations, and a number of technical and interpretive questions remain.[6-8] However, an example might demonstrate some of the potential of topographic brain mapping.

The 12-year-old child whose maps are produced in Figs 5 and 6 presented to a learning disorders program with a history of aggressive outbursts. His early development was relatively normal. A year prior to this evaluation while riding his bike he was struck by a motorcycle. The accident caused severe head injury, loss of consciousness, and a seizure. He had a left temporoparietal comminuted skull fracture and a left-sided epidural hematoma. A frontotemporal craniotomy was performed,

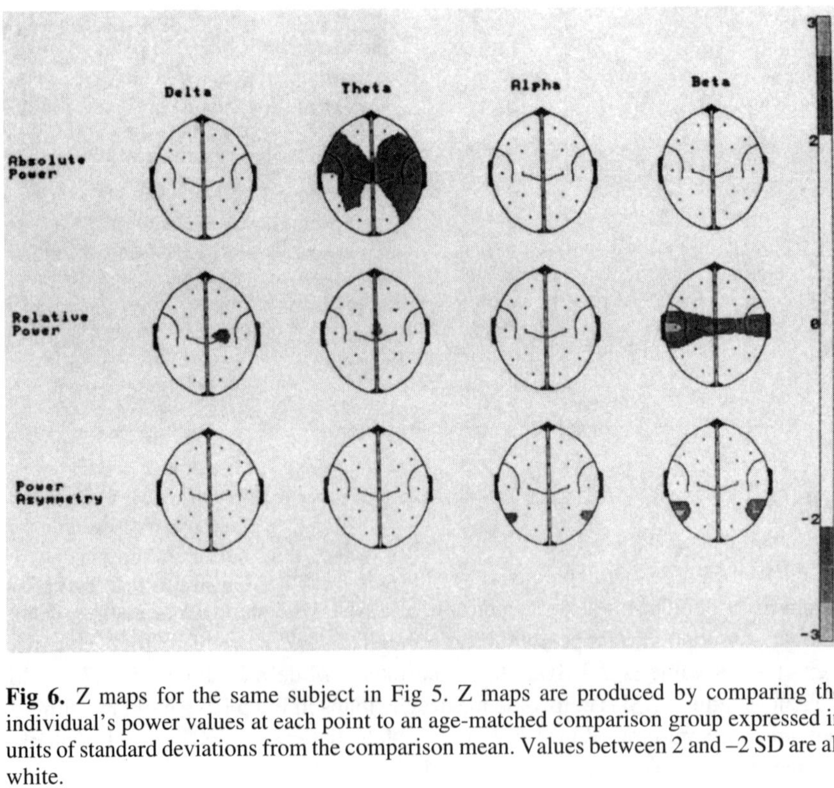

Fig 6. Z maps for the same subject in Fig 5. Z maps are produced by comparing the individual's power values at each point to an age-matched comparison group expressed in units of standard deviations from the comparison mean. Values between 2 and –2 SD are all white.

the hematoma was evacuated, and a small part of the damaged left anterotemporal lobe was removed. He recovered rapidly after the surgical procedure.

A year later his behavior was marked by rapid mood swings, tantrums and aggressive outbursts, short attention span, and distractibility. Neurologic evaluation of this left-handed child revealed a right-sided facial weakness, right-sided posturing on stressed gait, hyporeflexia of the left upper extremity, reduced strength in the left hand, left-sided synkinesias, and left somatosensory field neglect. Psychoeducational testing revealed a deficit in visuospatial processing, and a speech and language evaluation demonstrated difficulties with auditory memory but strong abilities with receptive and expressive language. Articulation was usually normal, but with fatigue his speech became temporarily hypernasal and indistinct.

One might be tempted to explain the right-sided neurologic abnormalities and the articulation problems by involving the damage to the left anterotemporal and left posterofrontal lobes. However, many left-sided neurologic abnormalities were noted as well, and his predominant learning disability appeared to be related to his deficits in visuospatial processing, both of which would be more likely explained by damage to the right temporoparietal area.

Topographic brain mapping of this child with a Z score transformation revealed a symmetric increase in absolute theta activity in the posterofrontal, anterotemporal, and anteroparietal areas, with a decrease in bilateral relative beta in the anterotemporal areas (Fig 6). Such a pattern might be seen with a contrecoup injury (an injury to the area of the brain opposite the primary point of impact due to the impact of the brain against the skull). An alternative explanation is that the damaged left temporal areas have been disconnected from the homologous right temporal areas, producing dysfunction in both areas. However, whatever the explanation, the topographic brain mapping appears to substantiate the finding of more extensive damage to brain function than originally anticipated and is consistent with the initially confusing findings on neurologic and psychoeducational evaluations. This patient has responded well to a regimen of methylphenidate and carbamazepine.

Evoked potentials

An evoked response or evoked brain potential is the brain's response to a specific stimulus. Approximately 100 ms after an auditory tone is presented, a negative polarity wave can be seen in the EEG tracing. However, often the amplitude of the voltage of that response is so low that it is buried in the ongoing EEG patterns. It is assumed that this "background" activity is unrelated to the stimulus, while the 100 ms deflection is a specific response to the stimulus. To better visualize the response, a number of stimuli are presented, are saved in the computer, then are averaged together. An average evoked response is the result (Fig 7).

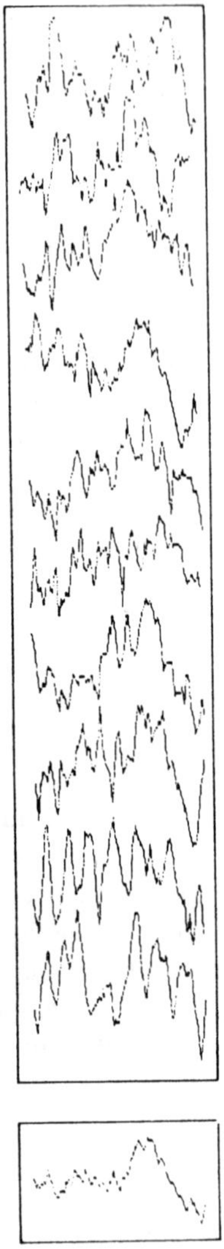

Fig 7. Averaged-evoked potentials. An averaged-evoked potential is produced by averaging the EEG response to many stimuli. Background noise tends to average to zero (because it is unrelated to the stimuli), while the evoked response emerges. In this example ten trials of EEG activity are presented (top), all starting exactly 75 ms prior to the auditory stimulus onset and continuing for 225 ms. The average of 20 stimuli is seen at the bottom. The negative wave peaking at approximately 160 ms (negative up) can also be seen in some of the raw traces. However, in most traces the background "noise" is equal to or greater than the evoked response and thus obscures it. The averaging process thus increases the signal-to-noise ratio.

If the same process is carried out at each electrode position, the voltage can then be plotted, instead of frequency or power (described above), to produce topographic maps. In the case of evoked potentials, the voltage is mapped rather than frequency or power, but the process is the same. The difference is that a series of maps is produced, one at each digitized point in time across a waveform.

Fig 8 demonstrates such an example in the study of the sensorimotor cortex of the premature infant. Somatosensory stimuli are used instead of visual or auditory stimuli because of the areas of the brain under study. Short, nonpainful electrical impulses are generated at the median nerve. The maps are the brain's response to those stimuli. Fig 8A reveals the map produced in response to bilateral median nerve stimuli, 184 ms, after the stimulus onset in a 32-week premature infant at 2 weeks of age. A symmetric, negative peak over the somatosensory cortex is clearly evident, with slight positivity more peripherally. The map of another premature infant with a bilateral grade 1 and a right-sided grade 4 intraventricular hemorrhage (IVH) and porencephalic cyst is seen in Fig 8B. If the map in Fig 8B is subtracted from the map in Fig 8A, a difference map is the result, indicating the focal nature of the IVH on the function of the somatosensory cortex. This can be compared to the CT scan in Fig 8D, which reveals the bilateral ventricular dilatation and right parietal porencephalic cyst. It is important to remember that the difference map in Fig 8C indicates an area of dysfunction in the map of the somatosensory evoked potential and does not necessarily always indicate the site of a structural lesion. However, it is precisely this dysfunction of normal brain physiology that mapping demonstrates. It is not an attempt to improve on the structural imaging capabilities that exist with CT and MRI scans.

Maps of the voltage of the evoked response are important to the study of the relationship between the brain and behavior, cognition and learning, because the evoked potential is a measure of the brain's specific response to a stimulus. As a result the evoked potential is dynamically related to the brain's processing of the information conveyed by the stimulus rather than the spontaneous background activity of the brain that is measured in the frequency maps that were described in the first part of this article.

Single electrode studies of simple stimuli such as flashes of light or pure-tone auditory stimuli reveal characteristic waveform peaks and as such are very important to the study of the integrity of the afferent sensory pathways. However, an even more exciting discovery is that even cognitive stimuli (requiring CNS processing, attention, or decision making), can produce characteristically different waves if the stimulus is relevant to a task that the subject must perform. Instead of tones, words presented verbally or visually can be used as the stimuli. If some of the words are correctly used in a sentence (eg, "The heart is red." and others are incorrectly used (eg, "The heart is yellow."), a negative wave will be produced in response to the incorrectly used words approximately 400 to 50 ms after the begin-

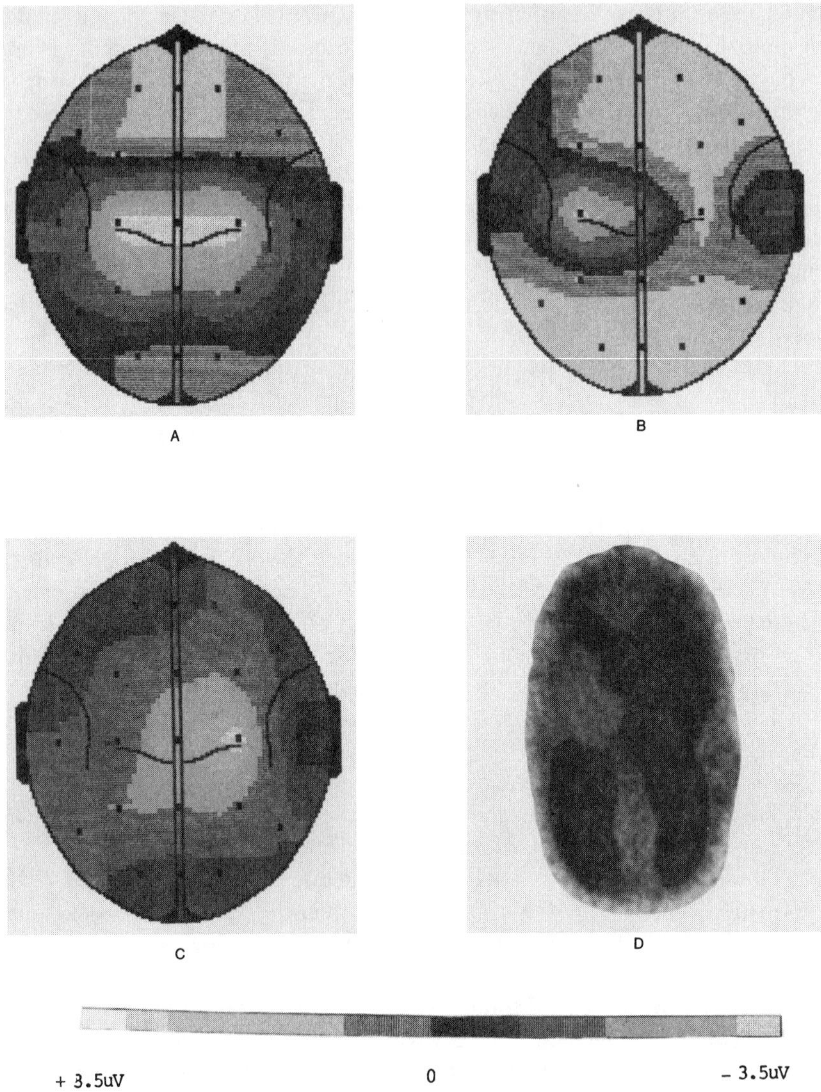

Fig 8. Evoked potential maps in intraventricular hemorrhage in a premature infant. **Fig 8A** is the map of a normal premature infant's response to bilateral somatosensory stimuli. A second infant with a grade 1 bilateral germinal matrix hemorrhage and a right hemisphere grade 4 hemorrhage and porencephalic cyst indicates the absence of the normal response in the right somatosensory area (**Fig 8B**). The difference map in **Fig 8C** indicates the area of functional differences. These maps can be compared to the CT scan, which reveals bilaterally dilated ventricles and the porencephalic cyst in the right parietal area (**Fig 8D**).

ning of the word, called the N400.[9] These waves are called event-related potentials rather than evoked potentials because they are dependent not on the characteristics of the stimulus itself but rather on the meaning of the stimulus to the subject at that point in time based on the task relevance of that stimulus to the subject.

Topographic mapping of these event-related potentials is now being actively studied in normal adults and in adults with specific neurologic and psychiatric disorders.[10-13] Although their use in children has been more limited,[14-16] they may prove very useful in the diagnosis and understanding of developmental disorders such as cerebral palsy, learning disabilities, and attention deficit disorder. For example, in one study children with reading disabilities were found to have reduced N400 amplitude compared to a normal comparison group.[17]

APPLICATION, POTENTIAL, AND LIMITATIONS

The group at the Brain Research Laboratories of New York University Medical Center has made the most extensive and systematic study of these techniques in a clinical population to date.[2,3,18-21] Using a specific approach to quantitative EEG called neurometrics, large samples of normal adults and adults with psychiatric disorders have been studied. Through a number of studies, characteristic topographic patterns have been described for patients with unipolar depression, bipolar depression, alcoholism, schizophrenia, mild cognitive impairment, and dementia.[18] Using the collapsed groups of normal adults—primary depression, alcoholism, and dementia—it was possible to correctly classify the subjects 72% to 80% of the time, depending on the disorder. When only unipolar and bipolar depressed patients were studied alone, differentiation accuracy was 85%. In a separate study in children,[19] four groups were studied; normal children, learning-disabled children with low IQs (65 to 84), learning disabled children with low-average IQs (above 85), and children with known neurologic disorders (eg, cerebral palsy, severe mental retardation, renal disease, and epilepsy). This group also consisted of children at risk with emotional disturbances and learning disabilities. Rather than attempting to classify the children into their correct group, neurometrics was used to make a judgment of normal or abnormal. Correct classification ranged from a low of 47% for the learning-disabled children with low-average IQs to a high of 89% for the children with known neurologic disorders.

Duffy and Als[14(p183)] studied infants, but because selection of the 11 infants was by referral from private pediatricians or pediatric neurologists because of "a minor suspicion of abnormality," few conclusions can be drawn about the ability of brain mapping to discriminate etiologic features in infants.

There are two serious problems with current clinical mapping studies that preclude their application to clinical populations. The group at the Brain Research Laboratories has been careful to use sophisticated statistical techniques to extract the most meaningful information from its extensive databases. While the group's ability to correctly classify adults with psychiatric disorders is impressive, it must be remembered that the same discriminating power will not be seen in clinical practice. The group's studies are designed such that each subject fits into a limited number of preestablished clinical categories (schizophrenia, bipolar depression, etc). Other patients with less typical features of a disorder, patients with rarer disorders, or patients with unknown entities are excluded. Because the atypical patient cannot fit into any of these preestablished categories, he or she will either be misclassified into an inappropriate diagnostic category or will be misidentified as normal. As the number of atypical cases in a population increases, the accuracy of prediction will decrease.

A second problem with clinical mapping studies is the heterogeneity of the groups. The Brain Research group describes its specific learning-disabled group as follows: "These children had no known neurological diseases but had IQ scores above 85 on the WISC-R and WRAT standard scores below 90 in language and/or arithmetic skills."[19(p178)] Although this definition may define a group of clinically similar children, it in no way assumes the same etiology. This is not to diminish the importance of these initial studies. They clearly break new ground in the objective assessment of children with learning and developmental problems. However, before they can be applied for widespread clinical use, more studies of objectively defined, homogeneous groups of children will be necessary.

This new technique for studying the topography of the brain's electrical activity is both promising and provocative. Only a few years ago production of the black and white contour maps required large computers and teams of software developers and engineers who were available in only a few of the more sophisticated experimental laboratories. Today the maps displayed in this article can be easily produced by an array of relatively inexpensive microcomputers. However, although these maps can be produced with relative ease, they must be viewed with great caution. The interpretation of topographic maps is hampered by a number of factors. For example, eye movements and activity from the muscles over the scalp produce artifacts that are often difficult to separate from the electrical activity produced by the brain.[22] Another important problem is that a peak of electrical activity produced at a specific electrode does not necessarily indicate that the brain structures underlying that electrode are responsible for the peak.[23-24]

In careful, skeptical hands, topographic mapping and quantitative EEG may be of great assistance to the clinician. In addition, these techniques, if studied with homogeneously defined populations and with appropriate experimental design, may provide the clinician with very valuable tools in the future for studying abnormal development in infants and children. However, the danger is that individuals without the appropriate knowledge will too readily draw unwarranted conclusions, thus exposing their patients to unnecessary and costly tests that yield pretty pictures but that do not affect patient care in the long run.

REFERENCES

1. Gevins AS: An overview of computer analysis, in Gevins AS, Remond A (eds): *Methods of Analysis of Brain Electrical and Magnetic Signals: EEG Handbook.* Amsterdam, Elsevier Science, 1987, pp 31–75.
2. Ahn H, Prichep L, John ER, et al: Developmental equations reflect brain dysfunctions. *Science* 1980;210:1259–1262.
3. John ER, Ahn H, Prichep L, et al: Developmental equations for the electroencephalogram. *Science* 1980;210:1255–1258.
4. Duffy FH, Bartels PH, Burchfield JL: Significance probability mapping: An aid in the topographical analysis of brain electrical activity. *Electroencephalogr Clin Neurophysiol* 1981;51:455–462.
5. Thatcher RW, Walker RA, Giudice S: Human cerebral hemispheres develop at different rates and ages. *Science* 1987;236:1110–1113.
6. Chiappa KH: Progress in topographic mapping of neurophysiological data: Comments, in Duffy FH (ed): *Topographical Mapping of Brain Electrical Activity.* Boston, Butterworths, 1986, pp 393–396.
7. Tyler HR: Progress in topographic mapping of neurophysiological data: A Critique, in Duffy FH (ed): *Topographical Mapping of Brain Electrical Activity.* Boston, Butterworths, 1986, pp 397–400.
8. Duffy FH: Brain electrical activity mapping: Issues and answers, in Duffy FH (ed): *Topographical Mapping of Brain Electrical Activity.* Boston, Butterworths, 1986, pp 401–417.
9. Kutas M, Hillyard SA: Reading senseless sentences: Brain potentials reflect semantic incongruity. *Science* 1980;207:203–205.
10. Duffy FH, Albert MS, McAnulty G: Brain electrical activity in patients with presenile and senile dementia of the Alzheimer's type. *Ann Neurol* 1984;16:349–448.
11. Morihisa JM, Duffy FH, Wyatt RJ: Brain electrical activity mapping (BEAM) in schizophrenic patients. *Arch Gen Psychiatry* 1983;40:719–728.
12. Morstyn R, Duffy FH, McCarley RW: Altered topography of EEG spectral content in schizophrenia. *Electroencephalogr Clin Neurophysiol* 1983;56:263–271.
13. Morstyn R, Duffy FH, McCarley RW: Altered P300 topography in schizophrenia. *Arch Gen Psychiatry* 1983;40:729–734.
14. Duffy FH, Als H: Neurophysiological assessment of the neonate: An approach combining brain electrical activity mapping (BEAM) with behavioral assessment (APID), in Brazelton TB, Lester BM (eds): *New Approaches to Developmental Screening of Infants.* Amsterdam, Elsevier Science, 1983, pp 175–197.
15. Duffy FH, Denckla MB, Bartels PH, et al: Dyslexia: Regional differences in brain electrical activity by topographical mapping. *Ann Neurol* 1980;7:412–420.
16. Duffy FH, Denckla MB, Bartels PH, et al: Dyslexia: Automated diagnosis by computerized classification of brain electrical activity. *Ann Neurol* 1980;7:421–428.
17. Stelmack RM, Saxe BJ, Noldy-Cullum N, et al: Recognition memory for words and event-related potentials: A comparison of normal and disabled readers. *J Clin Exp Neuropsychol* 1988;10:185–200.
18. John ER, Prichep LS, Fridman J, et al: Neurometrics: Computer-assisted differential diagnosis of brain dysfunctions. *Science* 1988;239:162–169.

19. John ER, Prichep L, Fridman J, et al: Neurometric evaluation of brain electrical activity in children with learning disabilities, in Duffy FH, Geschwind N (eds): *Dyslexia: A Neuroscientific Approach to Clinical Evaluation.* Boston, Little, Brown, 1985, pp 157–186.
20. John ER, Prichep L, Ahn H, et al: Neurometric evaluation of cognitive dysfunctions and neurological disorders in children. *Prog Neurobiol* 1983;21:239–290.
21. John ER, Karmel BZ, Corning WC, et al: Neurometrics. *Science* 1977;196:1393–1410.
22. Karson CN, Coppola R, Morihisa JM, et al: Computed electroencephalographic activity mapping in schizophrenia: The resting state reconsidered. *Arch Gen Psychiatry* 1987;44:514–517.
23. Lehmann D, Skrandies W: Spatial analysis of evoked potentials in man—a review. *Prog Neurobiol* 1984;23(3):227–250.
24. Lehmann D: Spatial analysis of EEG and evoked potential data, in Duffy FH (ed): *Topographical Mapping of Brain Electrical Activity.* Boston, Butterworths, pp 29–62.

Universal infant hearing screening and intervention: The Rhode Island Program

Richard L. Clarkson, PhD
Rhode Island School for the Deaf
Providence, Rhode Island

Betty R. Vohr, MD
Director, Neonatal Follow-up Program
Women and Infants' Hospital of Rhode Island
Brown University
Providence, Rhode Island

Peter M. Blackwell, PhD
Principal
Rhode Island School for the Deaf
Providence, Rhode Island

Karl R. White, PhD
Professor of Psychology and Special Education
Utah State University
Logan, Utah

ALTHOUGH EVERYONE agrees that children with hearing loss should be identified as early as possible,[1] currently available procedures in the United States have shown limited success in identifying the majority of hearing impaired children in their first year of life. In fact, recent findings by the Commission on Education of the Deaf[2] as well as the Academy of Otolaryngology—Head and Neck Surgery[3] indicate that the average age at which significant hearing loss is identified is 2½ years or greater. Even more alarming is the estimate that only 3% of the children born in the United States participate in any type of newborn hearing screening.[4] Given the critical importance of the first 3 years of life to all aspects of development, including speech, language, academic, social, and emotional aspects, a delay in identification or intervention is extremely detrimental and thus is not acceptable.

This broad range of developmental importance of newborn hearing screening is further emphasized in the *Healthy People 2000* report recently issued by the Department of Health and Human Services[5(p460)]:

> The future of a child born with a significant hearing impairment depends to a very large degree on early identification (ie, audiological diagnosis before 12 months of age) followed by immediate and appropriate intervention. If hearing impaired children are not identified early, it is difficult, if not impossible, for many of them to acquire the fundamental language, social and cognitive skills that provide the foundation for later schooling and success in society.[6–9] When early identification and intervention occurs, hearing impaired children make dramatic progress,

---

The work reported in this article was supported in part by project MCJ-495037, which was funded by the Maternal and Child Health Program (Title V, Social Security Act), Health Resources and Services Administration, United States Department of Health and Human Services, and by the Office of Special Education and Rehabilitation Services, United States Department of Education.

Inf Young Children 1994; 6(3): 65–74

> are more successful in school, and become more productive members of society. The earlier intervention and habilitation begins, the more dramatic the benefits.[2,10]

As important as early identification is, it is of little use if appropriate intervention programs are not initiated as soon as possible after the hearing loss has been identified. By coordinating the early identification and intervention programs, it is possible to significantly decrease the age at which hearing impaired children receive intervention, thus enhancing the overall provision of services. Following these assumptions, this article describes how the Rhode Island Hearing Assessment Program (RIHAP) addresses these two critical factors. Specifically, it discusses the implementation of statewide universal hearing screening of newborns by using a recently developed technology, the measurement of transient evoked otoacoustic emissions (TEOAE) and then describes the establishment of a follow-up system for delivering appropriate intervention services to infants identified with hearing loss.

The incidence of congenital, bilateral, severe-to-profound sensorineural hearing loss in the general population has typically been assumed to be between 1 and 2 infants per 1,000.[11-13] Recent research suggests that if all degrees of hearing loss, including mild and unilateral losses, are included, the prevalence may be 6 infants per 1,000.[14,15] Even if the lower rate is accepted, the prevalence of sensorineural hearing impairment is still significantly higher than the prevalence for other diseases for which screening is routinely done, such as phenylketonuria (PKU; 0.07/1,000), hypothyroidism (0.17/1,000), and sickle cell anemia (0.20/1,000).[16] When recurrent conductive hearing loss is included, the prevalence is substantially higher. The fact that the prevalence of hearing loss among newborns is so much higher than many other diseases for which infants are routinely screened is only one part of the argument for universal newborn screening. Just as important is the fact that early intervention is effective in ameliorating the negative consequences of congenital hearing loss by improving communication development in the child, reducing stress in the family, and ultimately reducing the eventual cost of special education services.[2,5,10]

WHY ALTERNATIVE METHODS OF HEARING SCREENING HAVE NOT BEEN SUCCESSFUL

Although considerable effort has been expended to identify infants and young children with hearing loss at an early age, most currently used screening procedures are either too expensive to implement or are not broad enough in their scope to successfully reduce the average age of identification. The four most prominent methods that have been used for hearing loss screening are behavioral testing in the home,[17-19] audiologic assessment of infants who are at high risk for hearing loss,[20,21] use of the Crib-O-Gram,[22] and use of auditory brain-stem response

(ABR).[23–26] Because none of these methods has proven successful for mass screening, the age of identification has not been significantly reduced in recent years.

For example, behavioral testing in homes is effective in countries where home visits are done routinely. But in countries such as the United States, the cost would be prohibitive. High-risk factors were once viewed as a mechanism for identifying most hearing impaired children, especially after the number of risk factors was updated and expanded.[27] Although children who exhibit one of these risk factors are more likely to be hearing impaired, approximately half of hearing impaired children never exhibit any of these risk factors.[28,29] Thus even if high-risk registry identification programs are perfectly implemented, they still miss most infants and young children with significant hearing loss. The Crib-O-Gram, a hospital-based alternative that records and correlates infant movement with predetermined emitted sounds, was seen as a promising alternative. But data on the validity of such techniques have been disappointing, as it is relatively ineffective in identifying infant hearing loss.[30]

Finally, the use of ABR in infants has been widely accepted as an accurate and objective methodology. Indeed this has contributed substantially to the American Speech-Language-Hearing Association's (ASHA) recommendation of ABR as the preferred method for screening infants' hearing. However, ABR screening is expensive, requires considerable training for administration and interpretation, and requires placement of electrodes on the head, which may be disturbing to the infant's state and uncomfortable for the parent. These factors may have led to ASHA's recommendation that ABR screening only be done with infants who exhibit one or more of the Joint Committee's 10 risk factors.[31] Unfortunately the present high-risk factors miss half of the hearing impaired infants. Thus ABR screening of high-risk infants would not successfully identify enough infants with hearing loss.

HEARING SCREENING TECHNIQUES USING TEOAEs

The problems noted with each of the most widely used screening techniques for early identification of hearing loss have probably contributed to the lack of success in substantially reducing the average age at which hearing impaired children are identified. However, the recent development of techniques to measure TEOAE promises significant progress in lowering the age of identification for children with hearing loss. TEOAEs, first described by Kemp,[32] are acoustic responses associated with the normal hearing process. Briefly, as sound enters the ear canal, it strikes the tympanic membrane and is transmitted through the middle ear's ossicular chain to the cochlea in the inner ear, where thousands of frequency-specific hair cells vibrate in a traveling wave to transmit the signal through the eighth cranial nerve to the brain. Kemp[32] showed that these hair cells simultaneously emit sound, or an "echo," back through the middle ear that can be measured with a low-noise microphone placed in the external ear canal.

Substantial evidence now shows that TEOAEs are a property of the healthy, normal-functioning cochlea, generated by active, frequency-selective, nonlinear elements within the cochlear partition. Further research shows that TEOAEs are *not* present in adults or children with hearing loss greater than 30 dB HL.[33–35] Consequently several researchers have suggested that TEOAEs may be a valuable, noninvasive, objective tool for evaluating cochlear status in infants and young children.[36–38]

Although the results from previous TEOAE research studies were promising, they were not compelling for several reasons: they all involved relatively small sample sizes; the majority of infants screened came from a neonatal intensive care unit (NICU); and the validity of the TEOAE technique was based on comparison with ABR results rather than on behaviorally confirmed hearing assessment. RIHAP, therefore, was designed to evaluate the feasibility, validity, and cost-efficiency of using TEOAEs as a universal newborn hearing screening technique and to use the existing service network to ensure early and appropriate intervention for infants and young children identified by the screening program. Detailed reports of the results of that evaluation are contained elsewhere.[14] The purpose of this article is to summarize the newborn hearing screening results and to describe how the screening program is integrated with the early intervention program.

THE RHODE ISLAND HEARING ASSESSMENT PROGRAM

RIHAP began in February 1990 as a cooperative venture between the Rhode Island School for the Deaf and Women and Infants' Hospital of Rhode Island (WIHRI) in conjunction with the Brown University Program in Medicine. While the establishment of a statewide hearing screening program was the major goal, RIHAP also sought to determine if a relatively new screening technique, the measurement of TEOAEs, could be used feasibly and cost-efficiently in screening large numbers of full-term and high-risk infants for hearing loss.[14,39]

Newborn hearing screening was done initially at WIHRI, a tertiary care center with an annual delivery rate of 9,200 infants. WIHRI has a 60-bed NICU, a 12-bed convalescent care nursery, 3 well-baby nurseries, and an alternative birthing suite. The Rhode Island School for the Deaf was included as a partner in the program because it was already providing educational programs to hearing impaired children, throughout the entire state of Rhode Island, a free audiologic clinic, and a statewide screening program of school-aged children. The cooperation between these institutions and the Department of Health was a crucial factor in the successful implementation of this project.

The multidisciplinary project planning team consisted of a pediatrician, an audiologist, educators, and a psychologist, who worked together to develop the study design, screening protocols, and study procedures. Prior to the initiation of the hospital-based screening, a training program emphasizing the importance of hearing screening was conducted for all hospital personnel involved with the program, including full-time medical staff, house officers, materials management personnel, medical records staff, and infection control staff. In addition, a personal letter was sent to every practicing pediatrician and family practice physician in the state describing the new screening program, and a hospital grand rounds was held on the topic. A brochure on hearing screening, which was developed specifically for parents, was included in the hospital preadmission packet and was placed in each infant's bassinet after screening. This brochure contained a simple, straightforward explanation of hearing screening and summarized the language development milestones parents should watch for as their baby became older.

The project staff currently includes a medical director, director of audiology, clinical audiologist, screening coordinator, screening technicians, clerical staff, and volunteers. Initially screening "teams" were established, which included a nurse, an audiologist, and a paraprofessional technician. At the end of the first year it was clear that paraprofessional technicians were fully capable of doing all screening and that the audiologist was better used to interpret the TEOAE data and to make recommendations concerning diagnostic evaluations. Specific screening protocols were developed and integrated into an operational system that was compatible with general hospital procedures. An ongoing process for monitoring the procedures of all screeners for adherence to the screening protocols was also implemented.

The screening coordinator is responsible for the daily operation of the program, including arranging work schedules, acting as a liaison to hospital personnel, and maintaining a management information and tracking system. The coordinator is knowledgeable about hearing impairment and resources within the community and is adept at facilitating the use of those resources. The director of audiology supervises all audiologic aspects of the project. She works with the clinical audiologist to monitor screeners, interpret screening results, and ensure that appropriate diagnostic audiologic assessments are completed for the identified infants. The audiologists maintain communication with a network of community audiologists throughout the state who provide follow-up diagnostic audiologic services. This permits each family to have access to the audiologist of its choice.

EQUIPMENT AND PROCEDURES FOR TEOAE

The ILO88 Otodynamics Analyzer, which is connected to an IBM compatible microcomputer and printer, is used to measure whether an infant has TEOAEs. A TEOAE screening takes approximately 10 minutes per infant for screeners who are skilled with the equipment and comfortable in handling infants. Although contemporary hospital practices have resulted in shorter stays for full-term infants, recent research suggests that delaying screening until just prior to discharge improves the pass rate, as it provides more opportunity for debris in the external ear canal to clear naturally.[40,41] Thus there is a slightly lower pass rate for infants who are less than 24 hours of age when screened.

The actual screening process involves three basic stages.[40] First, the infant must be in a quiet state with a properly fitted probe so that an adequate stimulus can be reliably presented. Next, the test is run and the screener evaluates several aspects of the testing situation to determine if the test was valid. If technical problems associated with any of these areas are identified, they are corrected, and the testing is repeated. Finally, test results are scored by the audiologist to determine whether to pass the infant or to refer him or her for further testing. Examples of the testing results of an infant who passed and of one referred for further evaluation are shown in Fig 1. The information in the upper right-hand corner in the "Response FFT" box of each result shows whether there is an emission (the clear area) present above the background noise. As can be seen, the "pass" has an emission, but the "refer" does not.

RESEARCH DESIGN TO EVALUATE THE VALIDITY OF TEOAE SCREENING

To evaluate the validity of measuring TEOAEs as a newborn hearing screening technique, a prospective clinical trial involving 1,850 infants was initiated at WIHRI. A complete summary of this research is reported by White et al.[14] In brief, the study design, shown in Fig 2, included two samples of infants. The first consisted of 464 infants screened with both TEOAE and auditory brain-stem response (ABR) regardless of the test results. This was done so that comparisons could be made between the two procedures. The second sample consisted of 1,386 infants who were screened initially with TEOAE and were only screened with ABR if they failed the TEOAE. Those infants who failed either one of the screening tests were brought back to the hospital 4 to 6 weeks later for a second-stage TEOAE and ABR screen. After the second-stage screening, infants who did not pass were referred for a diagnostic ABR test or a behavioral audiologic evaluation. Details of the screening procedures are given by Johnson et al.[39]

DESCRIPTION OF INTERVENTION FOR INFANTS WITH HEARING LOSS IDENTIFIED DURING SCREENING

The efficacy of screening programs is ultimately determined by the successful entry of children with hearing loss into appropriate intervention programs. RIHAP, in conjunction with the Family Guidance Program at the Rhode Island School for the Deaf, and the Rhode Island Department of Health's early intervention system, has developed a statewide service network for infants identified as having a hearing loss. Infants with significant hearing loss identified by the screening program and their families were referred to the service network for com-

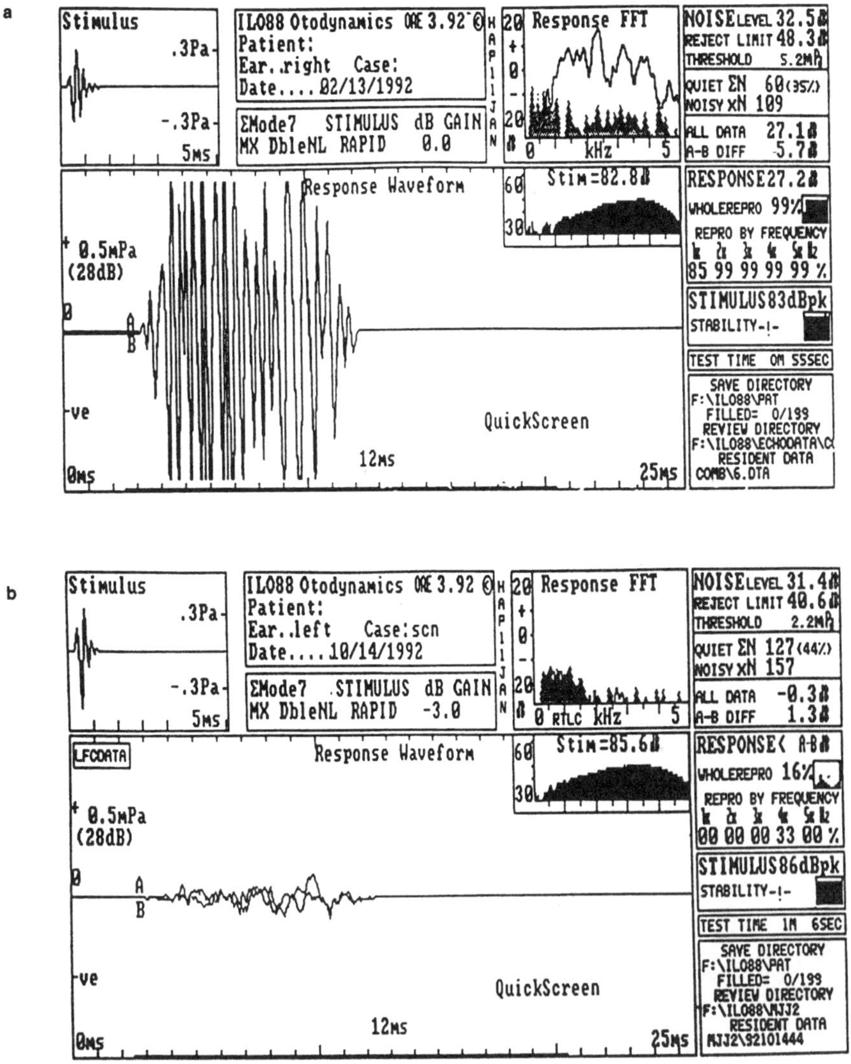

Fig 1. Examples of results for transient evoked otoacoustic emission (TEOAE) screening for (a) neonate with normal hearing, and (b) a neonate who did not exhibit an emission.

prehensive audiologic, medical, and communication services as mandated by Public Law 99-457. The Family Guidance Program provided family-centered services to families of infants and toddlers with moderate to profound sensorineural hearing loss. These services were designed to assist parents during the critical times associated with the identification of a hearing loss.

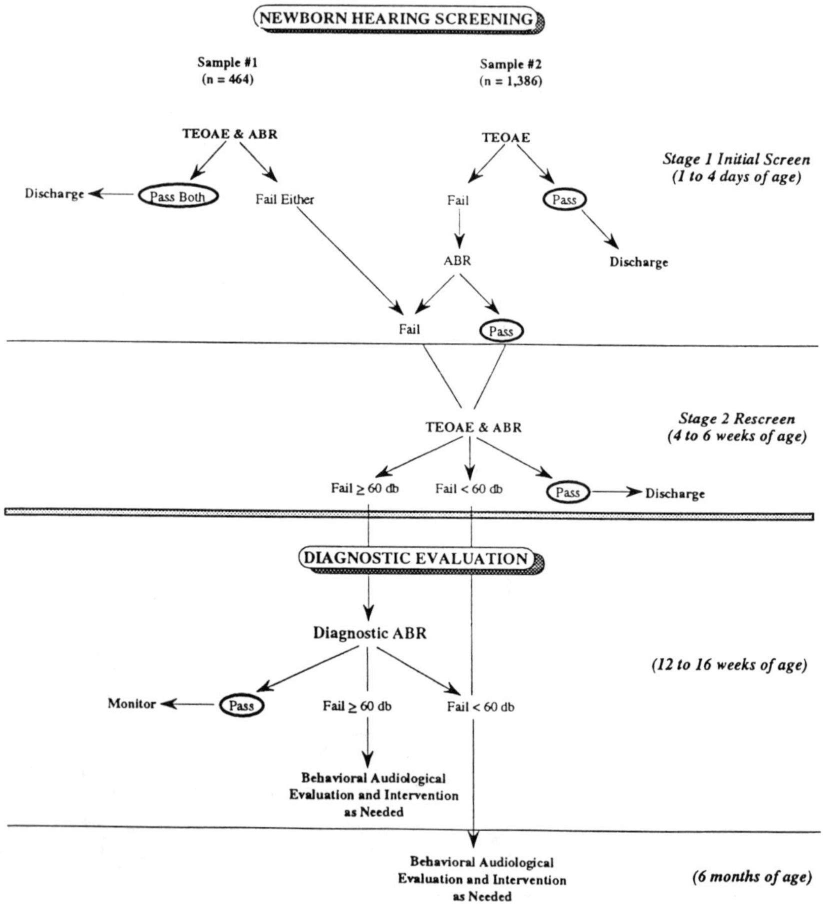

Fig 2. Design for prospective clinical trial of TEOAE screening. Reprinted with permission from *Seminars in Hearing.* 1993;14(1):21. Thieme Medical Publishers, Inc.

Program staff included a team of audiologists, speech and language specialists, teachers, social workers, and psychologist who worked together to provide a variety of services. All aspects of communication development, carried out in settings appropriate for the child's developmental level and hearing loss, were emphasized. Training formats included individual sessions, structured language activities for the parent and child, small play groups for preschool, and home-bound programs. Audiologic management assisted parents in making decisions about amplification, in integrating auditory skills into daily activities, and in monitoring middle ear function with pediatric or otolaryngology referral when indicated.

The program also provided emotional support to the family as they coped with the child's hearing loss. Individual sessions, support groups, workshops on topics of interest, and classes in sign language were offered. At the same time, parents were assisted in processing the wide range of information that accompanied the knowledge that their young child was hearing impaired. Parents were guided through the many important decisions that needed to be made at this critical time and were helped with referrals for other services and with transition planning as the child approached the age of 3 years and became eligible for educational services in the local community through an individualized education plan (IEP).

Infants with milder degrees of hearing impairment have typically been identified at a later age and present different kinds of needs. Recent research, however, now demonstrates that unless appropriate early intervention is provided, these children experience substantial deficits in speech/language development and in academic and social skills.[42,43] For these children, many of whom have unilateral sensorineural or recurrent conductive hearing losses, their delays are often more subtle. Thus the above-mentioned services needed to be modified.

Intervention for children with mild sensorineural and recurrent conductive losses focused on assisting parents in getting appropriate audiologic and medical services for their child, monitoring speech and language development so that more direct intervention could be provided if delays began to emerge, and teaching parents how to modify their normal activities with the child to stimulate language development and to use appropriate communication techniques to compensate for whatever level of hearing loss their young child was experiencing. A more complete explanation of the services needed by such children is given by Brackett et al.[44] RIHAP also provided regular tympanometric and otologic management, communication assessment and follow-up, and parent education. Other services to these families were provided in conjunction with one of the state's other early intervention programs and used the Family Guidance Program at the School for the Deaf for consultation purposes.

RESULTS OF NEWBORN HEARING SCREENING

Of the 1,850 infants included in the initial cohort of the clinical trial, 115 (6.2%) were referred for further diagnostic evaluation following the two-stage screening process. Eighty-four of the 115 referrals (73%) received a complete audiologic evaluation, including behavioral assessments in every case. Results of the evaluations indicated that 11 of the infants had sensorineural losses and 37 had recurrent conductive losses (operationally defined in this study as having hearing thresholds of greater than 25 dB HL and abnormal tympanograms on 2 or more behavioral, audiologic evaluations separated by at least 4 weeks). Of the 11 infants with sensorineural hearing losses, 6 had bilateral, severe-to-profound losses; 4 had unilateral, severe-to-profound losses; and 1 had a unilateral moderate loss.[14] This suggests an overall prevalence of sensorineural loss of 5.95 per 1,000; 2.59 per 1,000 in the normal nursery; and 23 per 1,000 in the NICU. Four of the 11 infants did not have any high-risk factors identified by the Joint Commission on Hearing. Thus in hearing screening programs that only screen infants with risk factors, these infants would have been missed.

The average age of identification (ie, confirmed hearing loss based on audiologic evaluation) for the 11 children with sensorineural hearing loss was 5.5 months. This is substantially lower than the national average of 30 months.[2,3] In each case appropriate intervention programs were made available to the family shortly after the hearing loss was identified.

DISCUSSION

The purpose of the study was to evaluate the feasibility, validity, and cost-efficiency of integrating a TEOAE-based universal newborn hearing screening program with a statewide network of services. Data from an initial cohort of almost 2,000 infants clearly demonstrate that the technique is fast, simple, and feasible for hospital-based, universal screening. Second, the results confirm and extend those from previous research in demonstrating that TEOAE is extremely accurate in identifying both sensorineural and recurrent conductive hearing losses. Finally, a detailed cost analysis reported elsewhere shows that the two stages of newborn hearing screening cost about $25 per infant screened,[45] thus making it economically viable.

Beyond the above research findings lie the broader conclusions that universal infant hearing screening and follow-up intervention can be accomplished and that the Rhode Island Hearing Assessment Program provides a model of implementation for other states. While each state must establish a program based on its unique resources and needs, the present project reflects the recent recommendations of the National Institute of Health Consensus Development Conference.[15] The consensus panel, being aware of the significant implication of hearing loss on a child's development, concluded that all infants should be screened for hearing impairment, not just high-risk infants. It further recommended that the first screening should be done by measuring OAEs because it is quick, inexpensive, and accurate. Furthermore, the panel recommended follow-up testing with ABR, followed by a comprehensive hearing evaluation no later than 6 months.

Since September 1992, every live birth at Women and Infants' Hospital (approximately 65% of the births in the state) has been screened. By December 1993, infant hearing screening will be completed on every newborn in the state. Infants who are screened and determined to have a hearing loss will be referred immediately for early intervention. As this and other projects develop, further improvements in efficiency are expected such that the age of identification and intervention will decrease significantly. The success of RIHAP is based not only on the use of an effective hearing screening method but on a cooperative network involving hospitals, pediatricians, early intervention teams, audiologists, schools, and parents. RIHAP began as a multidisciplinary team effort and continues as a statewide multidisciplinary program for infant screening and family service provision.

REFERENCES

1. Northern JL, Downs MP. *Hearing in Children.* 3rd ed. Baltimore, Md: Williams & Wilkins; 1984.
2. Commission on Education of the Deaf. *Toward Equality: Education of the Deaf.* Washington, DC: US Government Printing Office; 1988.
3. American Academy of Otolaryngology—Head and Neck Surgery. Infant hearing screening program launched. *Bull Am Acad Oto Head Neck Surg.* 1990;9:46–47.
4. Bess FH, Hall JW. *Screening Children for Auditory Function.* Nashville, Tenn: Bill Wilkerson Center Press; 1992.
5. US Department of Health and Human Services. *Healthy People 2000: National Health Promotion and Disease Prevention Objectives.* Washington, DC: Public Health Services; 1990.
6. Coscarelli-Buchanan JE. Finding ears that do not hear. *J Tenn Med Assoc.* 1986;79:39.
7. Lyon DJ, Lyon ME. Early detection of hearing loss. *Can J Pub Health.* 1982;73:410–415.
8. Riko H, Hyde ML, Alberti PW. Hearing loss in early infancy: incidence, detection, and assessment. *Laryngoscope.* 1985;95:137–145.
9. Riko H, Hyde ML, Corgin H, Fitzhardinge PM. Issues in early identification of hearing loss. *Laryngoscope.* 1985;95:373–381.
10. Coplan J. Deafness: ever heard of it? Recognition of permanent hearing loss. *Pediatrics.* 1987;79:206–213.
11. Fitzaland RE. Identification of hearing loss in newborns: results of eight years' experience with a high-risk register. *Volta Rev.* 1985;87:195–203.
12. McCormick B, Curnock DA, Spavins F. Auditory screening of neonates using the auditory response cradle. *Arch Dis Child.* 1984;59:1168–1172.
13. Bergman I, Hirsch RP, Fria TJ, Shapiro SM, Holzman I, Painter JJ. Cause of hearing loss in the high-risk premature infant. *J Pediatr.* 1986;106:95–101.
14. White KR, Vohr BR, Behrens TR. Universal newborn hearing screening using transient evoked otoacoustic emissions: results of the Rhode Island Hearing Assessment Project. *Semin Hear.* 1993;14(1):18–29.
15. NIH Consensus Development Conference. Summary of the NIH Consensus. Bethesda, Md: Office of Medical Applications of Research; March 1993.
16. Batshaw ML, Perret YM. *Children with Handicaps: A Medical Primer.* Baltimore, Md: Brookes Publishing; 1981.
17. Barr B. Early identification of hearing impairment. In: Taylor IG, Markides A, eds. *Disorders of Auditory Function, Vol III.* New York, NY: Academic Press; 1980.
18. Bentzen O, Jensen JH. Early detection and treatment of deaf children: a European concept. In: Gerber SE, Mencher GT, eds. *Early Management of Hearing Loss.* San Francisco, Calif: Grune & Stratton; 1981.
19. McCormick B. Hearing screening by health visitors: a critical appraisal of the distraction test. *Health Vis.* 1983;56:449–451.

20. Mahoney TM, Eichwald JG. Model program V: a high-risk register by computerized search of birth certificates. In: Swigart ET, ed. *Neonatal Hearing Screening.* San Diego, Calif: College Hill press; 1986.
21. Schuler V, Rushmer N. *Parent-Infant Habilitation: A Comprehensive Approach to Working with Hearing-impaired Infants and Toddlers and Their Families.* Portland, Ore: Infant Hearing Resource Publications; 1987.
22. Miller K, Simmons FB. A retrospective and an update in the Crib-O-Gram neonatal screening and follow-up: clinical trials. Seminar presented at the annual meeting of the American Speech-Language-Hearing Association. November 1984. Atlanta, Ga.
23. Galambos R, Despland PA. The auditory brainstem response (ABR) evaluates risk factors for hearing loss in the newborn. *Pediatr Res.* 1980;14:159–163.
24. Kilney PR. New insights on infant ABR hearing screening. *Scan Aud.* 1988;30:81–88.
25. Levi H, Tell L, Feinmesser M, Gafni M. Sohmer H. Early detection of hearing loss in infants by auditory nerve and brainstem responses. *Audiology.* 1983;22:181–188.
26. Murray AD, Jave E, Watson CS. Prognostic validity of auditory brainstem evoked response screening in newborn infants. *Am J Otolaryngol.* 1985;6:120–131.
27. Joint Committee on Infant Hearing. 1990 position statement. *ASHA.* 1991;33(5):3–6.
28. Elssmann SF, Matkin ND, Sabo MP. Early identification of congenital sensorineural hearing impairment. *Hear J.* 1987;40:13–17.
29. Mauk GW, White KR, Mortensen LB, Behrens TR. The effectiveness of screening programs based on high-risk characteristics in early identification of hearing impairment. *Ear Hear.* 1991;12:312–319.
30. Shimizu H, Walters RJ, Kennedy DW, Allen MC, Markowitz RK, Luebkert FR. Crib-O-Gram vs. auditory brainstem response for infant hearing screening. *Laryngoscope.* 1985;95:806–810.
31. American Speech-Language-Hearing Association. Guidelines for screening for hearing impairments and middle ear disorders. *ASHA.* 1990;32(2):17–24.
32. Kemp DT. Stimulated acoustic emissions from within the human auditory system. *JASA.* 1987;64:1386–1391.
33. Bray P, Kemp DT. An advanced cochlear echo technique suitable for infant screening. *Br J Aud.* 1987;21(2):191–204.
34. Kemp DT, Bray P, Alexander L, Brown AM. Acoustic emission cochleography—practical aspects. In: Cianfrone G, Grandori F, eds. *Cochlear Mechanics and Otoacoustic Emissions.* Stockholm, Sweden: Almquist & Wiskell Periodical; 1986.
35. Probst R, Lonsbury-Martin BL, Martin GK, Coats AC. Otoacoustic emissions in ears with hearing loss. *Am J Otolaryngol.* 1987;8:71–73.
36. Bonfils P, Uziel A, Pujol R. Screening for auditory dysfunction in infants by evoked otoacoustic emissions. *Arch Oto Head Neck Surg.* 1988;114:887–890.
37. Lutman ME, Mason SM, Sheppard S, Gibbin KP. Differential diagnostic potential of otoacoustic emissions: A case study. *Audiology.* 1989;28:205–210.
38. Stevens JC, Webb HD, Hutchinson J, Connell J, Smith MF, Buffin JT. Evaluation of click evoked otoacoustic emissions in the newborn. *Br J Aud.* 1991;25:1–14.
39. Johnson MJ, Maxon AB, White K, Vohr BR. Operating a hospital-based universal newborn hearing screening program using transient evoked otoacoustic emissions. *Semin Hear.* 1993;14(1):46–56.

40. Vohr BR, White KR, Maxon AB, Johnson MJ. Factors affecting the interpretation of transient evoked otoacoustic emission results in neonatal hearing screening. *Semin Hear.* 1993;14(1):57–72.
41. Kok MR, VanZanten GA, Brocaar MP, Wallenburg HCS. Click-evoked otoacoustic emissions in 1036 ears of healthy newborns. *Audiology.* 1993;32:213–224.
42. Teele DW, Klein JO, Rosner BA. Otitis media with effusion during the first three years of life and development of speech and language. *Pediatrics.* 1984;74:282–287.
43. Clarkson RL, Eimas PD, Marean GC. Speech perception in children with histories of recurrent otitis media. *JASA.* 1989;85(2):926–933.
44. Brackett D, Maxon AB, Blackwell PM. Intervention issues created by successful universal newborn hearing screening. *Semin Hear.* 1993;14(1):88–104.
45. Johnson JL, Mauk GW, Takekawa KM, Simon PR, Sia CCJ, Blackwell PM. Implementing a statewide system of services for infants and toddlers with hearing disabilities. *Semin Hear.* 1993;14(1):105–118.

Understanding children with chronic lung disease. Part I: Lung function

Clint Swanson, Jr, MA, RRT
Senior Pediatric Respiratory Therapist
Department of Respiratory Care
Kluge Children's Rehabilitation Center and Research Institute

Mark A. Brown, MD
Assistant Professor
Department of Pediatrics
University of Virginia Health Sciences Center
Charlottesville, Virginia

RECENT TECHNOLOGIC advances have drastically increased the survival rate of infants with severe, life-threatening illness. These complex infants and children have filled our long-term care facilities to capacity and caused an outflow into the community. The pediatric intensive care units of the past are now located within our homes, and we have been forced into special care practices. This type of care requires both active and assertive intervention to improve outcome, especially for children with chronic lung disease.

This series of articles provides a brief look at normal and abnormal pulmonary (lung) conditions in an effort to raise the comfort level of interdisciplinary caregivers (therapists, teachers, etc) and to ensure that normal interactive treatment sessions are attained. It is divided into two parts. Part I, "Lung Function," describes normal lung anatomy and physiology and introduces the reader to some of the more common disorders affecting lung function in infants and young children. Part II, "Respiratory Supports and Treatments," follows this section.

CLINICAL RESPIRATORY PHYSIOLOGY

Upper respiratory tract

The primary function of the upper airways (Fig 1) is to filter, warm, and humidify inspired air. By the time it reaches the throat, inspired air at room temperature is warmed to approximately 86°F and moistened to 80% relative humidity. This is accomplished largely by three parallel shelflike projections in the nose called the turbinates. The turbinates separate air flow into smooth streams, increasing mucous membrane contact and thereby facilitating maximal humidity and heat transfer. Additional soft tissues and narrow nasal passages severely reduce the space available for nasal air flow in the young pediatric population. Infants are also obligate nose breathers, that is, they rely almost exclusively on their nasal passages when breathing. These anatomic and functional differences cause what would be mild cold symptoms in the adult to result in major airway discomfort for the infant.

The authors would like to thank Tami Brown for assistance in manuscript preparation and Joy Everhart, RN, for preparation of the figures.

Inf Young Children 1992; 5(2): 68–77

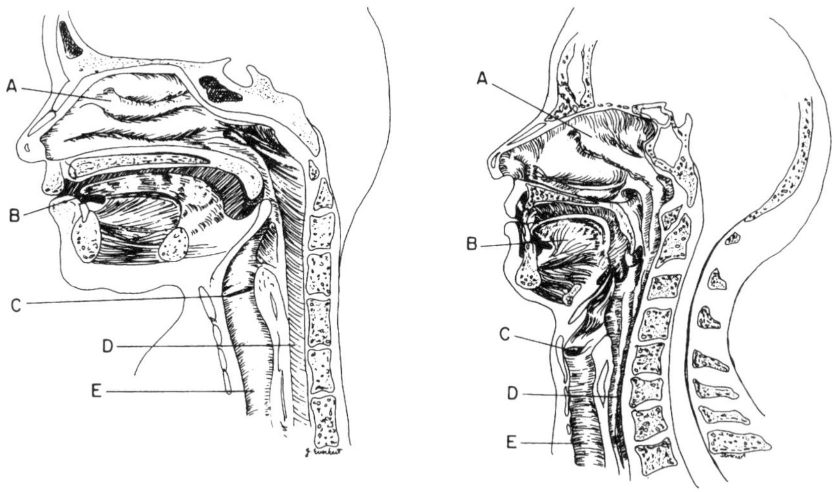

Fig 1. Comparison of upper airway anatomy of the adult (left) and young child (right) showing the turbinates (A), tongue (B), larynx (C), esophagus (D), and trachea (E).

The infant larynx (voice box) is more flexible and is positioned upward and forward compared to that of the adult. It enables speech production, prevents foreign matter from entering the trachea (windpipe), and can aid breathing by producing grunting on expiration. Grunting creates a back pressure to help keep the alveoli (air sacs) open and promote oxygenation.

Lower respiratory tract

Although smaller in all dimensions, the lower airways of the infant and child are nearly identical to those of the adult (Fig 2). Smaller airway diameters of the trachea, bronchi, and bronchioles (the smaller airway branches) lend themselves to greater resistance to the movement of air into and out of the lungs. Similar degrees of airway edema (swelling of the lining of the airways) cause critical reductions in air flow in infants but only minor changes in the adult. These changes in the pediatric patient may be evident by flaring (opening outward) of the nostrils, which is an attempt to make the airway larger and to reduce the resistance to air flow. The more flexible chest wall of the infant responds to the increased efforts to breathe by collapsing. This increased effort can also lead to a sucking inward (or retraction) of the skin above the clavicles or between the ribs or an inward movement of the sternum (breastbone). Infants and young children normally have a more rapid respiratory rate than adults. It is typically around 40 breaths per minute in the

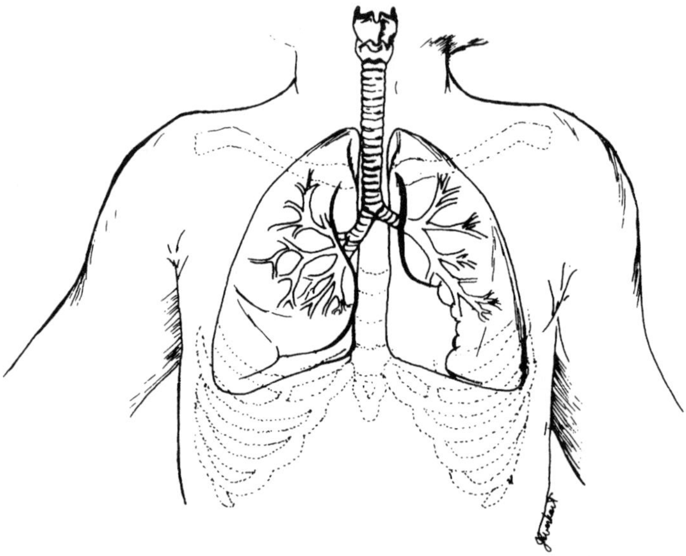

Fig 2. Diagram of the lower respiratory tract from just below the larynx, showing sequential branching, which creates smaller and smaller airways.

newborn and may increase significantly in infants with chronic lung disease and/ or respiratory tract infection.

Circulation

Unoxygenated blood flows from the body through the right side of the heart to the lungs and returns to the left side of the heart to be pumped throughout the body. Blood flow in the lungs is regulated by the response of the blood vessels to acid level and oxygen. A decrease in respiration leads to a build-up of carbon dioxide and a decrease in oxygen, which in turn increases acid levels in the blood and alveoli. This causes constriction of the blood vessels within the lung and a corresponding increase in pulmonary (artery) blood pressure. Increased pulmonary artery pressures increase the workload on the right side of the heart and can cause right-sided heart failure in children with chronic lung disease.

Under normal conditions pulmonary blood flow (perfusion) is relatively evenly matched to gas exchange (ventilation). Any condition that reduces lung ventilation (eg, infection or smoke inhalation) will cause ventilation/perfusion mismatching and will decrease blood oxygen levels. Heart and lung functions are therefore closely related and require careful monitoring in children with chronic pulmonary disease.

Natural defenses against disease

Normal clearance mechanisms exist to protect the tracheobronchial tree from foreign matter and disease-causing organisms. In addition to laryngospasm (constriction or closure of the voice box to prevent entry of foreign matter into the lungs), a continuous mucous blanket lines the lung and functions to capture inhaled debris. Mucus is propelled out of the lung by tiny cilia, hairlike projections that rhythmically beat and promote continuous upward movement of mucus. These mechanisms, combined with continuous air flow during breathing, promote mucus clearance.

The newborn protects its airway through reflexive sneezing, the only functional airway clearance mechanism in early infant development. During the first few weeks of life, the cough reflex develops to become the primary means of airway drainage when the cilia and mucous blanket fail. Cough is elicited by stimulation of cough receptors in the ear canals, trachea, and smaller air passages.

Another type of defense is provided by the immune system, which releases antibodies to combat invading viruses and bacteria on the inside surfaces of the lungs. Defense is also carried out by large cells that engulf and digest foreign matter and bacteria.

CONTROL OF BREATHING

Central control

The brainstem (pons and medulla) controls the unconscious regulation of rhythmic breathing (Fig 3). Special cells called chemoreceptors, which are sensitive to changes in acid levels within the fluid surrounding the brain (cerebrospinal fluid, CSF), lie within the brainstem. Carbon dioxide rapidly diffuses between blood and CSF. Thus, an increase in blood acidity (caused by increased levels of carbon dioxide) translates to a corresponding increase in acid level. The central chemoreceptors respond by sending a signal to the respiratory system to rid the body of excess carbon dioxide. This is the principal mechanism for respiratory control.

Peripheral control

Other chemoreceptors, located in the wall of the carotid arteries of the neck and the aorta (the main blood vessel of the body), are sensitive to decreases in blood oxygen. These peripheral chemoreceptors have many small blood vessels themselves and consume oxygen faster than any other tissue within the body. Thus, when blood oxygen levels drop, these receptors immediately sense the change, stimulate the brainstem to activate increased respiration, and promote an increase in heart rate. These chemoreceptors are also responsive to acid levels and carbon

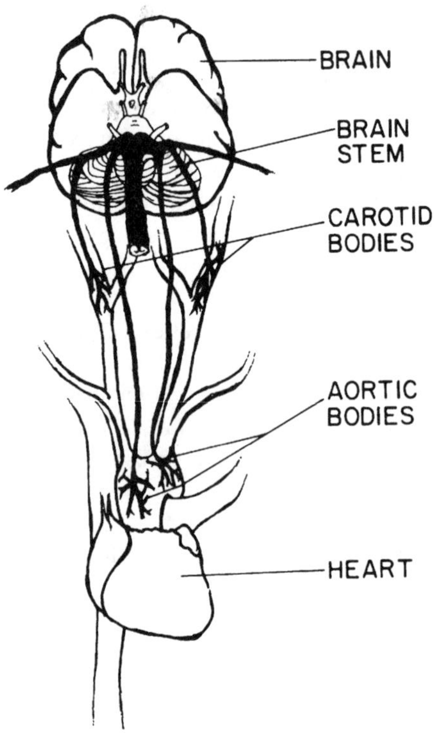

Fig 3. Schematic of the peripheral chemoreceptors (carotid and aortic bodies) and their connection with the brainstem.

dioxide, but to a much lesser degree. Therefore, hypoxemia (decreased oxygen in the blood) is a secondary stimulus to respiration. In the case of chronic respiratory failure (chronically increased carbon dioxide levels), oxygen levels in the blood become the primary control mechanism for breathing because the body has become accustomed, and therefore unresponsive, to higher carbon dioxide levels.

Alteration of control

The normal breathing pattern is the product of a complex excitatory and inhibitory control system. Total system integrity (brain and chemoreceptors) must be present for balance. Injury or certain drugs may interrupt either excitatory or inhibitory networks within the brain or chemoreceptors and will upset this delicate balance, causing irregular breathing or apnea (absence of spontaneous breathing).

MECHANICS OF AIR EXCHANGE

The primary muscle for breathing is the diaphragm (Fig 4). It is actually composed of two muscles, the left and right hemidiaphragms, which separate the chest and abdominal cavities. These muscles are stimulated by the phrenic nerve and act as the bellows or pump for breathing. Intercostal muscles (muscles between the ribs) act to lift and push outward the front ribs. This forces air in and out by changing the diameter of the chest. Additional, or accessory, muscles such as the sternocleidomastoid, trapezius, scalene, and pectoralis operate to assist the diaphragm during periods of increased breathing effort, such as exercise or severe respiratory illness. The intercostal and other accessory muscles are not normally activated during resting breathing.

Generation of air flow

Inhalation is the result of contraction of the diaphragm, which creates an increase in chest volume and negative pressure within the chest cavity (Fig 4). Air

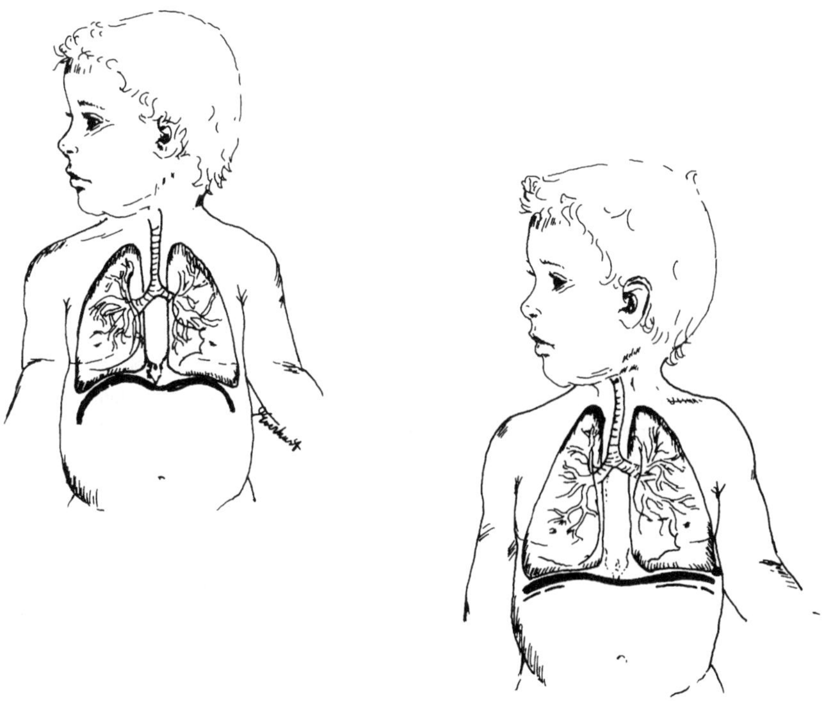

Fig 4. Changes associated with inspiration including descent and flattening of the diaphragm and expansion of the lungs.

flows from the mouth (high pressure) to the alveoli (low pressure). Exhalation, on the other hand, is normally a passive process brought about by muscle relaxation. It can be enhanced by active participation of the intercostal and abdominal muscle groups during periods of increased respiratory effort in response to exercise or blocked air passages.

Work of breathing (WOB) is closely related to the resistance to air flow within the lungs. A small reduction in airway size results in a large decrease in the cross-sectional area of the airway, a marked increase in airway resistance, and a dramatic increase in WOB. WOB is also related to lung compliance (distensibility). Like a new balloon, the lungs are more difficult to expand in infancy but become more compliant with age. After adolescence, however, they grow increasingly resistant to distention throughout adulthood. The infant chest wall, lacking stability as previously stated, is less able to overcome situations of increased resistance (eg, infection) or decreased compliance (eg, bronchopulmonary dysplasia) and collapses with increased WOB. Other signs of increased WOB include tachypnea (increased respiratory rate), retractions (use of accessory muscles), and nasal flaring.

Volumes, capacities, and forces

Tidal volume is the amount of air inhaled or exhaled during quiet breathing. Minute ventilation is the amount of gas moved into or out of the lungs in 1 minute and is calculated by multiplying tidal volume by the respiratory rate. Vital capacity is the total amount of air that can be drawn in after a maximal expiration or exhaled after a maximal inspiration. Vital capacity is one of the most important indicators of pulmonary reserve. Unfortunately, clinical signs of respiratory distress do not show up until it is severely diminished.

One respiratory force measurement, the negative inspiratory force, bears mention because it relates to the amount of muscle force generated in taking a deep breath. It is used often in conjunction with vital capacity as a measure of respiratory muscle strength in patients with neuromuscular diseases. The measurement of tidal volume and negative inspiratory force is highly dependent on technique, clinician expertise, and the activity level/emotional state of the patient. Vital capacity measurements are further dependent on patient cooperation, which is rarely available in the birth to 3-year age group. Bedside volumes and forces are rough screening tools only and should never be used as absolute measurements to guide treatment.

Components of respiration

Ventilation

Ventilation is quite simply the movement of gas into and out of the lungs. It is directly related to respiratory rate, tidal volume, and whether the lungs have an increase in compliance (distensibility) or resistance in regard to air flow. Ventilation directly affects the amount of carbon dioxide in the blood and therefore the blood acid level. A feedback loop exists to increase respiratory rate and/or tidal volume when an increase in carbon dioxide level is detected by either central or peripheral chemoreceptors. The subsequent decrease in carbon dioxide then leads to a return to normal respiratory rate and/or tidal volume.

Oxygenation

As with carbon dioxide, gas must be moved into and out of the alveoli for oxygen to be taken up by the blood. The oxygen concentration of the inspired air (fraction of inspired oxygen, FiO_2) also affects oxygen concentration in the blood. Air contains approximately 21% oxygen. Any increase in FiO_2 increases the tendency for oxygen to diffuse across the lung surface into the blood. Oxygenation also depends on the number of red blood cells available to bind with oxygen and the thickness of the membrane between the air and the blood.

Changes in pulmonary blood flow can drastically alter the amount of oxygen in the blood. If the time that red blood cells have to pass by alveoli and gather oxygen (oxygen binds to the hemoglobin molecule on the red blood cell) is significantly decreased, there is less time for oxygen to enter the bloodstream. If ventilation/perfusion mismatching occurs (some areas receive blood but not ventilation, while others receive ventilation but not blood), blood is not exposed to oxygen, which therefore decreases the total blood oxygen level.

Delivery of oxygen to tissues

Oxygen must bind to hemoglobin in the red blood cells and circulate through the body for tissue oxygenation to occur. When a hemoglobin molecule binds to oxygen, it is said to be saturated. Oxyhemoglobin saturation (percentage of hemoglobin molecules bound to oxygen) is an indirect measure of the amount of oxygen available to the tissues. An oxyhemoglobin saturation of 90% or greater is normal. Lung injury can affect all aspects of oxygenation except FiO_2 and hemoglobin content. Hence oxygenation problems can often be overcome by increasing the concentration of inspired oxygen or increasing hemoglobin with a blood transfusion.

Disease states and how the lungs compensate

Restrictive lung disease is characterized by a loss of lung and/or chest wall compliance, which makes the lungs stiff and difficult to expand. Vital capacity and tidal volume measurements may be reduced. Infants compensate for reduced air flow by breathing faster (tachypnea). Bronchopulmonary dysplasia is an example of a restrictive lung disease.

Obstructive lung disease is manifest by an increased resistance to air flow through the airways. Residual volume (the amount of air remaining in the lungs after exhaling) is increased because of air trapping, leaving less lung available for moving air in and out. Asthma is a form of obstructive lung disease. Compensatory mechanisms include tachypnea initially with a progression to accessory muscle use, retractions, head bobbing (up and down head movements with respiratory efforts), and nasal flaring as the obstructive process worsens.

Decreased oxygenation can initially be corrected by tachypnea alone. As oxygen levels in the blood are further decreased, grunting may be necessary to normalize blood oxygen levels by recruiting more alveolar units through the creation of back pressure, as explained earlier.

All compensatory mechanisms serve to maintain normal net ventilation of the lungs by increasing the amount of air going into the lungs or by maximizing the lung surface exposed to air through the recruitment of alveolar units by grunting. They do so, however, at the cost of increased effort and therefore energy expenditure, which over time may exhaust the infant and/or utilize calories normally devoted to growth.

DISORDERS ASSOCIATED WITH ALTERED PULMONARY STATUS

There are a number of disorders that may lead to abnormal respiratory function in the infant and young child. We have somewhat arbitrarily divided them into those disorders resulting from abnormalities present at birth (congenital disorders) and those disorders resulting from an injury or insult after birth (acquired abnormalities). All these disorders result in restrictive lung disease, obstructive lung disease, or both, and they are often accompanied by decreased oxygenation.

Congenital disorders

Malacia

The larynx and the large and medium-size airways depend upon the presence of firm, well-formed cartilage for their structural integrity. If this cartilage fails to develop properly, the structure involved may be floppy, resulting in various degrees of obstruction to air flow. This floppiness, or malacia, may occur at the level of the larynx box (laryngomalacia), within the trachea (tracheomalacia), or in the large or medium-size bronchi (bronchomalacia). It may also occur in combination. If the abnormality lies outside the chest—that is, laryngomalacia or tracheomalacia involving the portion of the trachea that lies within the neck—the obstruction to air flow occurs during inspiration and results in a medium- or high-pitched sound during inspiration called stridor. Laryngomalacia and tracheomalacia involving that portion of the trachea outside the chest rarely are severe enough to lead to life-threatening obstruction of air flow. In these cases, however, tracheostomy may be required to bypass the area of obstruction.

If the abnormality involves an airway lying within the chest, the obstruction to air flow occurs during exhalation, often manifesting as a chronic cough that typically is mild to moderate in severity. In the vast majority of cases the abnormal cartilage becomes firmer with time, and most patients recover fully by 6 to 12 months of age.

Fistula

During normal development, the trachea and esophagus begin as a single tube that pinches off to form two separate tubes. Rarely, a connection between the two remains intact and is called a tracheoesophageal fistula. Although in most cases this can be corrected surgically, there is often abnormal cartilage in the area of the fistula, leading to some degree of malacia. From a functional standpoint, this is nearly identical to tracheomalacia as described above. It may, however, take longer than the usual 6 to 12 months to resolve and may never fully correct itself.

Congenital syndromes

There are a number of well-described congenital syndromes, some associated with chromosomal abnormalities, that are associated with altered airway anatomy. Some of these are listed in the box. These may be associated with abnormalities in the structure of the nose, mouth, or throat that can lead to obstruction of air flow. If abnormalities of the respiratory centers of the brain are involved, there may also be abnormal control of breathing. In some cases, there may be abnormal functioning of the muscles of the mouth and throat, leading to disordered swallowing. Constant leakage or aspiration of saliva or food into the lungs leads to pneumonia, recurrent lung injury, and chronic lung disease.

Chest wall abnormalities

As previously discussed, the chest wall must be relatively rigid for the respiratory muscles to work efficiently. Deformities of the chest wall, either in isolation or as part of a constellation of congenital abnormalities, may decrease the efficiency of the respiratory muscles and lead to restrictive lung disease.

Congenital Syndromes Associated with Altered Airway Anatomy

Beckwith-Wiedemann syndrome
CHARGE association
Cleft lip and palate syndrome
de Lange's syndrome
Möbius sequence
Robin sequence (Pierre Robin syndrome)
Treacher Collins syndrome
Trisomy 18

Asthma

Asthma, sometimes referred to as reactive airways disease, is a disease characterized by intermittent reversible obstruction to air flow secondary to muscular spasm in the airways, swelling of the lining of the airways, and an increased production of airway secretions in response to a number of stimuli[1] These abnormalities increase the resistance to air flow, increase WOB, and, when severe, can be life threatening. Symptoms may be brought on by colds; noxious stimuli such as cigarette smoke, paint, or solvent fumes; or, in some cases, agitation. Asthma is treated with bronchodilators (eg, theophylline and albuterol) and corticosteroids (anti-inflammatory medications). It is unusual for uncomplicated asthma to be severe enough in infants to debilitate them to the point of necessitating rehabilitation. It is, however, often a significant component of bronchopulmonary dysplasia (described later) or cystic fibrosis.

Cystic fibrosis

Cystic fibrosis (CF) is the most common lethal genetically transmitted disease among Caucasians, occurring in 1 of every 2000 births.[2] In the United States, 1 in 20 individuals or 5% of the population carries the gene for CF.[2] Although carriers for CF are normal, people with the disorder have an abnormality of the cells lining the respiratory and gastrointestinal tracts, leading to chronic and recurrent pneumonia and difficulty with digestion, particularly digestion and absorption of fats. The lung disease is generally mild in infancy, but it can be quite severe and require oxygen, multiple medications, and frequent physiotherapy to promote drainage of secretions from the respiratory tract. With the isolation of the abnormal gene responsible for CF,[3] new and more specific treatments may be possible in the future.

Abnormal control of breathing

Abnormalities of the central nervous system may, through mechanical effects on the respiratory centers, lead to abnormal control of breathing. Rarely, this may occur without any detectable physical abnormality of the brain. Such children are said to have central hypoventilation or Ondine's curse. Respiratory efforts may often be normal when the child is awake, only to become abnormal or even cease during sleep. These individuals are difficult to treat medically, often requiring tracheostomy and/or some form of mechanical ventilatory support during sleep.

Acquired respiratory tract abnormalities

Subglottic stenosis

In infants and young children who require the placement of an endotracheal tube into the trachea for respiratory support, scar tissue may develop. This most commonly occurs in the area just below the larynx and may lead to a significant narrowing of the trachea. This narrowing, or subglottic stenosis, may result in obstruction of air flow, which may be mild and of little consequence or severe enough to necessitate placement of a tracheostomy. Placement of an endotracheal tube may also lead to a localized malacia. This is rarely severe enough to warrant tracheostomy but may cause mild symptoms, usually stridor or cough.

Spina bifida

The spectrum of abnormalities included under the common name spina bifida (myelomeningocele), an abnormality of the development of the spinal column and spinal cord, may also be associated with respiratory problems. Most commonly, this is the form of abnormal control of breathing because of abnormalities of the brain and/or spinal cord that exert mechanical effects on the central respiratory centers. These children may also have difficulty swallowing properly (see below).

Abnormal swallowing

In some children, an injury to the central nervous system from lack of oxygen during birth (perinatal asphyxia), traumatic brain injury, or other insult may result in cerebral palsy with an associated abnormality of swallowing. This may also be associated with congenital syndromes (as previously discussed) or severe forms of muscle diseases, such as certain types of muscular dystrophy. The disorder in swallowing may lead to the chronic aspiration of oral secretions or food into the lungs, causing recurrent pneumonia and chronic lung damage.

Bronchopulmonary dysplasia

Bronchopulmonary dysplasia can be defined as a chronic lung disease requiring oxygen therapy in any infant older than 28 days who experienced respiratory failure from any cause requiring mechanical ventilation in the first 3 days of life.[4] It is characterized by asthmalike symptoms with increased lung resistance, decreased lung compliance, and some degree of diffusion block that decreases the ability of oxygen to enter the bloodstream. These abnormalities lead to increased WOB and increased oxygen consumption in the face of decreased oxygen uptake. It is often treated with oxygen, bronchodilators (medications that relax airway muscles), diuretics (medications to relieve excess fluid accumulation), and aggressive nutritional support. Because this disorder is common in premature infants, it often occurs simultaneously with developmental disabilities.

Other

Other abnormalities such as lung cysts, tumors within the chest, or abnormalities of lung development may result in abnormal pulmonary function. Many of these are surgically correctable and leave little in the way of significant permanent residual effects. In older children, scoliosis can be an important cause of restrictive lung disease. It is rarely a factor in the infant or young child.

• • •

The process of normal respiration is the result of the coordinated action of the muscles of respiration, particularly the diaphragm. It is controlled by the brainstem and monitored by special cells called chemoreceptors, which send signals to the brainstem to stimulate it to adjust the breathing pattern to maintain a normal balance of oxygen and carbon dioxide in the blood. Disease or injury may affect any portion of the respiratory system and elicit changes in the respiratory pattern in an attempt to compensate for the resulting impairment.

In "Understanding Children with Chronic Lung Disease. Part II: Respiratory Supports and Treatments" various technologies and methods for assisting infants and young children with chronic lung disease to maintain normal or nearly normal respiratory function are discussed.

REFERENCES

1. American Thoracic Society. Standards for the diagnosis and care of patients with chronic obstructive pulmonary disease (COPD) and asthma. *Am Rev Respir Dis.* 1987;136:225–244.
2. Nadler HL, Ben-Yoseph Y. Genetics. In: Taussig LM, ed. *Cystic Fibrosis.* New York: Thieme-Stratton; 1984.
3. Rammens JM, Iannuzzi MC, Derem B-S, et al. Identification of the cystic fibrosis gene: chromosome walking and jumping. *Science.* 1989;245:1059–1065.
4. Bancalari E, Adenenour GE, Feller R, et al. Bronchopulmonary dysplasia: clinical presentation. *J Pediatr.* 1979;95:819–823.

Understanding children with chronic lung disease. Part II: Respiratory supports and treatments

Mark A. Brown, MD
Assistant Professor
Department of Pediatrics
University of Virginia Health Sciences Center

Clint Swanson, Jr, MA, RRT
Senior Pediatric Respiratory Therapist
Department of Respiratory Care
Kluge Children's Rehabilitation Center and Research Institute
Charlottesville, Virginia

IN PART I OF THIS two-part series about the care of young children with severe respiratory difficulties, a description of normal and abnormal lung function was presented. With that brief introduction to respiratory physiology and pathophysiology as a background, Part II will present an introduction to those devices used most commonly to provide support for children with chronic lung disease. It is hoped that this presentation will raise the comfort level of interdisciplinary caregivers (therapists, teachers, and so forth), so that more appropriate and effective interaction between those caregivers and the infant or child can occur. Guidelines for assessing whether or not an infant or child is in respiratory distress are also given, and safety concerns for both the child and caregiver are discussed.

ASSESSMENT: CLINICAL SIGNS OF RESPIRATORY DISTRESS

Respiratory rate

It can be very frightening to encounter an infant or child with a rapid respiratory rate. Infants and young children respond initially to increased carbon dioxide levels or decreased oxygen saturation by increasing their respiratory rate. It is the respiratory rate, in conjunction with the tidal volume, that produces the minute ventilation required to maintain homeostasis. Restrictive lung disease (a loss of lung or chest wall compliance) and obstructive lung disease (an increase in resistance to air flow) both manifest initially as an increase in respiratory rate or tachypnea. Thus, tachypnea may be an early sign of distress. It is important to remember, however, that other factors, such as activity and elevated body temperature, may also lead to an increased respiratory rate and that respiratory rate must be interpreted within the context of the overall condition of the infant or child. Table 1 lists age-specific respiratory rates in infants and young children.

The authors thank Tami Brown for assisting in manuscript preparation and Bo Read, RRT, of University Respiratory Care for providing the equipment used in the figures.

Inf Young Children 1993; 5(3): 57–66

Table 1. Mean respiratory rates of infants and young children

Age	*Awake**	*Asleep**
6–12 months	64 (58–75)	27 (22–31)
12–24 months	35 (30–40)	19 (17–23)
24–48 months	31 (23–42)	19 (16–25)

*Range is shown in parentheses.

Adapted with permission from Waring WW. The history and physical exam. In: Kendig, Cherniak, eds. *Disorders of the Respiratory Tract in Children.* Philadelphia, Pa: W.B. Saunders; 1983: 63.

Work of breathing

An increased respiratory rate, in light of acute illness or chronic disease, will increase carbon dioxide production and oxygen consumption. As work of breathing (WOB) is increased, other clinical manifestations such as flaring, retractions, or grunting may be observed. Flaring of the nostrils lowers upper airway resistance by enlarging airway diameter at the external naris. Retractions—a depression of the skin between the ribs, above the collarbones, or above the breast bone—occurs as lung compliance decreases and indicates the presence of increased effort to inspire. Grunting, a creation of back-pressure by the vocal cords to increase pressure in the lungs, also occurs when WOB is increased.

Any or all of these signs, in addition to an increased respiratory rate, can be found on assessing an infant or child with chronic lung disease. It is important that each caregiver become familiar with each individual patient's baseline respiratory pattern and rate in order to recognize acute changes indicative of distress.

Color

Cyanosis, a blue coloration of the skin, nail beds, or mucous membranes, occurs when there is insufficient oxygen in the blood. Peripheral cyanosis (acrocyanosis) occurs in the distal extremities and usually indicates a transient condition of reduced blood flow (perfusion), and not necessarily reduced blood oxygen levels. Progression to the central cyanosis, blueness of the mucous membranes of the mouth or tissues around the mouth, usually indicates advancing hypoxemia (reduced oxygen in the blood). This condition requires prompt attention on the part of the caregiver to assure adequate respiratory function. If present, supportive ventilation and oxygenation equipment should be checked for proper application and operation.

Breath sounds

Listening to the chest is important in determining the onset of respiratory distress in infants and young children with chronic lung disease. By familiarizing oneself with the routine sounds of the patient's chest the caregiver will be able to readily discern acute changes. Normal air flow may be restricted during inspiration and cause a crowing sound or stridor. Stridor may be caused by narrowing of the larynx or trachea from infection or stricture (scarring). Whether present or absent during resting respiration, stridor may become more noticeable during periods of agitation or crying. If it is not usually observed, it is a reason for medical concern and should be promptly evaluated by a physician.

Wheezing is a sound produced by the partial obstruction of small airways from mucus or bronchoconstriction (swelling and spasm within the bronchi or breathing tubes). Wheezing may be present in children with reactive airways disease, cystic fibrosis, or bronchopulmonary dysplasia (BPD). The onset of wheezing or an increase from baseline could indicate a worsening condition. Most patients will have nebulized medications already prescribed to treat chronic obstructive airway conditions. If wheezing is a new finding, if it steadily worsens, or if it is not remedied by nebulized medication treatment, it should be evaluated by a physician.

Grunting, as previously described, is another sound that can be heard in the chest. It generally indicates increased WOB and should be evaluated by a physician.

Any of the aforementioned changes from baseline are true indicators of acute distress in the patient with chronic lung disease. These changes in breath sounds, combined with respiratory rate, depth of breathing, nasal flaring, retractions, and sometimes temperature, can give the caregiver information that can lead to the early recognition of an impending respiratory exacerbation.

Physician-directed evaluation

Once the physician is notified, usually because the caregiver has noticed a change in the patient's baseline assessment, a diagnosis-directed evaluation is instituted to determine the cause and appropriate treatment. The physician may order an arterial blood gas to check blood acidity and carbon dioxide and oxygen levels or a chest radiograph to look for fluid in the lungs or congestion. Finally, laboratory studies may be ordered to check blood electrolytes, blood chemistry, or medication levels. Each of these tests, combined with a full physical assessment by the physician, are used to prescribe treatment.

SUPPORT TREATMENT

Chest physiotherapy

A wide variety of techniques is generally employed under the heading of chest physiotherapy. Clinically, chest physiotherapy usually indicates percussion applied to the chest to promote mucus clearance. Percussion, which involves clapping the chest with a cupped hand or rubber percussor, is a time-honored technique whose efficacy has recently come under scrutiny. Nevertheless, because many patients currently receive percussion, it is important to discuss the technique.

Percussion on the chest of the small infant and child must be done with great care. The caregiver must be aware of hand position (Fig 1) and the force used to clap the chest at all times. Percussion with a tightly cupped hand or percussor should never be applied over the external rib margins, lower breast bone (xiphoid), stomach, liver, spine, or kidneys. Percussion should be vigorously but comfortably applied over a towel or blanket to protect the skin. Vibration—shaking the hands vigorously while in contact with the chest—is also employed at each position to mobilize secretions. It is important that vibration only be applied to exhalation to ensure that adequate air flow, and thus shearing force, is realized at the airway wall.

Postural drainage (Fig 1), another form of chest physiotherapy, requires moving the patient into various positions to promote bronchial drainage by utilizing the force of gravity. Both percussion and postural drainage techniques should be ordered by the physician and taught by qualified nurses and therapists before being administered by family members or other caregivers. Percussion strength, vibration technique, percussion and postural drainage positions, and frequency of treatment are considered to be patient specific and disease specific in order to promote maximum effectiveness and comfort. The primary care physician should be consulted if questions or problems relative to therapy administration arise.

Incentive spirometry

Incentive spirometry is a useful technique with some children in the birth to 3 years of age group. Blowing games, soap bubbles, and pinwheels have been successfully used by many patients to improve vital capacity and respiratory strength and prevent atelectasis (collapse of alveoli). Success is contingent on patient rapport, understanding, and the degree to which the patient enjoys the treatment. Several flow and volume displacement devices are on the market for use as incentive spirometers. A highly structured, patient-specific selection process must be employed in order to assure correct choice of device.

Other techniques

Other techniques, such as positive expiratory pressure (PEP) and diaphragmatic exercises, have been used to promote mucus clearance and increase respiratory strength in the pediatric population. Although these techniques are most successfully employed in children who have reached the age of complex verbal understanding, they do have limited usefulness in the birth to 3 years of age group. PEP

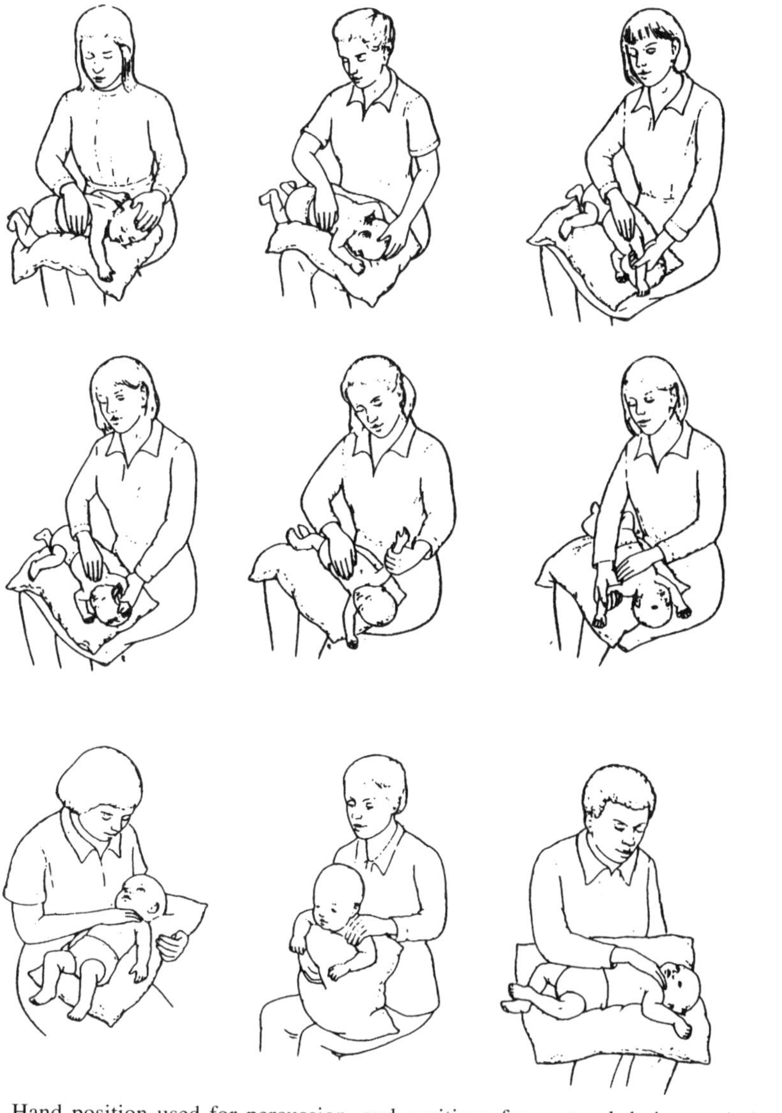

Fig 1. Hand position used for percussion, and positions for postural drainage. Artist: Dimitri Karetnikov.

applies 5 to 10 cm H_2O pressure at the mouth of a spontaneously breathing patient. This technique keeps positive pressure within the airway, prevents premature airway collapse, and prolongs expiratory flow, which promotes mucus mobilization. It is extremely important that a low deadspace apparatus be used in order to prevent the rebreathing of carbon dioxide from exhaled breath. A mask device can be used where voluntary lip closure cannot be achieved. It is important to note, however, that masks are not well tolerated in the young pediatric population, thus severely limiting the efficacy of PEP.

The efficacy of diaphragmatic exercises is limited to situations where diaphragmatic strength has been reduced and can be rehabilitated with externally applied resistive techniques (placement of weight on the abdomen of a child lying in a supine position). Confidence, comfort, and endurance should guide all exercise sessions. Diaphragmatic weight-to-body-weight ratios, repetition, and frequency are all specific to the patient and disease.

Humidification

Room humidifiers have been used for many years to add humidity to the inspired air. Close attention must be paid to the desired goal of the humidification before a device is chosen. Neither heated nor cool humidifiers offer any advantage in a well-ventilated room where the heating or cooling system causes frequent total air exchanges to occur. Relative humidity (moisture in the air) may be slightly increased in small, poorly ventilated spaces with either heated or cool room humidifiers. Cool humidity is much more soothing to the upper airways. Heated humidifiers are usually less apt to spread infection because of a hot element near the humidifier outlet. Both cool and heated room humidifiers must be routinely and thoroughly cleaned to prevent the growth of organisms that can cause disease.

Whenever the upper airways (nose and oropharynx) are bypassed, as with endotracheal and tracheostomy tubes, humidity must be applied or conserved to limit mucosal drying (drying of the lining of the lungs) and mucus inspissation. One device suited to humidity conservation (Fig 2) consists of a T-piece with two paper filters that absorb water vapor from the exhaled air and deliver it to the inspired breath. Although not completely efficient, this device can extend the time that a pediatric patient may be away from his or her humidifier, thus promoting normal play activities and improved developmental interventions. Another device (Fig 2) is available for use with ventilators to increase ventilator portability. Children wearing these devices must be closely supervised to prevent airway obstruction from mucus or fluid occlusion of the filter material or increased drying of secretions.

Relative humidity can best be increased by the direct application of a device (Fig 2) that applies heated or cool moisture to the airway. Direct application is accomplished through the use of various masks, hoods, and tents that physically connect the patient to the humidity apparatus. Most devices in respiratory care apply humidity (moisture you cannot see) or aerosol (water droplets) that are suspended in air or oxygen. Both types can be heated, if applied directly to the tra-

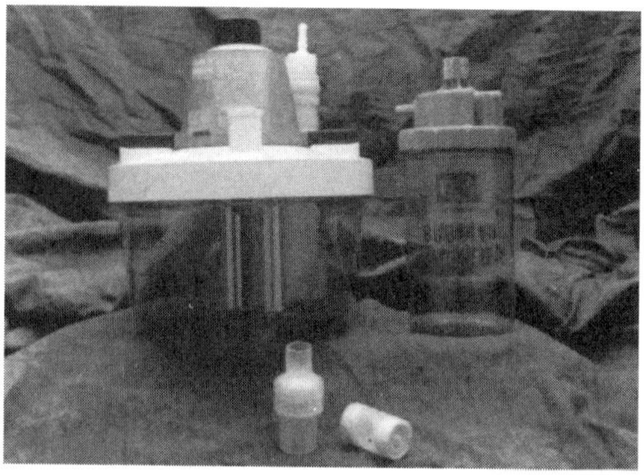

Fig 2. Humidification devices (clockwise from top left): heated "cascade" humidifier, bubble humidifier, "artificial nose" for application directly to tracheostomy tube, "artificial nose" for a home ventilator circuit.

cheobronchial tree, or cool, if applied to the upper airways. If the device uses a heat source, it must be maintained at near normal airway temperatures (approximately 30°C to 34°C) where it enters the patient.

OXYGEN THERAPY

Delivery devices

Most oxygen therapy devices can be divided into low-flow or high-flow systems. A low-flow system does not supply enough gas to meet total patient inspiratory demand. Therefore additional room air must be drawn in to make up the difference. A system of this type can administer any percentage of oxygen from 21% (room air) to greater than 90%. Low-flow systems are not very dependable, however, because inspired oxygen percentages can change with breathing rate and depth. Conversely, a high-flow system supplies enough gas to surpass inspiratory requirements and thus delivers a constant percentage of oxygen to the patient. This type of system can supply oxygen percentages between 21% and 100%.

The nasal cannula (Fig 3) is perhaps the most widely used device for low-flow oxygen administration. It is simple and well tolerated by infants and young children. Oxygen flow rates are generally titrated to keep oxygen saturation greater than 92%. Other devices such as the mask or face tent (Fig 3), although poorly tolerated by young pediatric patients, are employed when greater oxygen percentages are required. The tracheostomy collar (Fig 3), used to administer oxygen and humidity to patients with tracheostomy tubes, is generally employed as a high-flow system. Each caregiver should be familiar with individual patient care specifics in order to prevent excessive gas flow rates, especially in small infants.

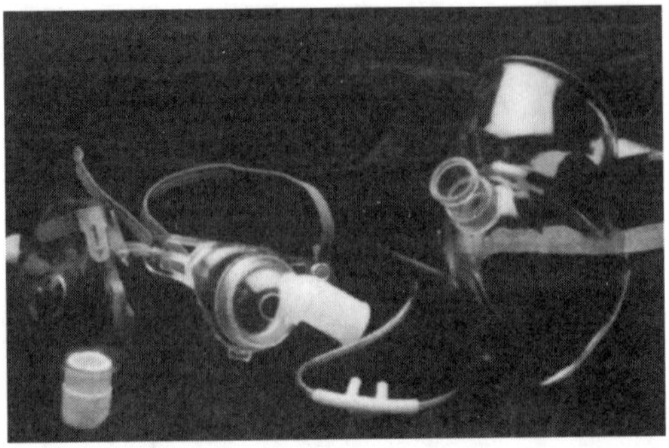

Fig 3. Oxygen administration devices (left to right): face mask, trach collar, nasal cannula, and face tent.

Delivery systems

Oxygen delivery systems are generally limited to compressed gas cylinders, liquid oxygen systems, and oxygen concentrators. Compressed oxygen cylinders range in weight and capacity from approximately 3 lb containing 75 L of oxygen to 135 lb containing 6,900 L. All compressed oxygen cylinders are painted green, employ a regulator to reduce tank pressure to 50 psi, and use a flow meter to deliver an accurate, controlled flow of oxygen to devices such as those previously discussed. Oxygen tanks are useful for periodic oxygen use, portability, and administration of low flow rates of oxygen. They are quite heavy and require frequent monitoring to assure that supply is not interrupted.

When larger amounts of oxygen are used, generally greater than 1 L/min for 24 hours a day, liquid and concentrator systems are superior to cylinders. Liquid systems use the low boiling point of oxygen (–297°F) and its tremendous expansion rate (1 cu ft of liquid oxygen expands to about 860 cu ft or about 28 L of gaseous oxygen) to deliver a continuous flow of oxygen from a small reservoir. Oxygen concentrators produce oxygen from room air (which is comprised of 78% nitrogen and 21% oxygen) by means of a molecular sieve. Room air is compressed and pushed through the sieve to trap oxygen and remove nitrogen. Concentrators, due to design, limit delivery to less than 100% oxygen. The percentage of oxygen delivered gas is inversely related to total flow settings; that is, higher flow rates deliver lower oxygen concentrations. This relationship is not usually of consequence in the young pediatric population due to the low flow rates that are utilized.

Humidification devices (Fig 2) are normally employed with oxygen delivery devices to prevent drying of mucous membranes and secretions. Cylinders, liquid oxygen systems, and, under certain circumstances, oxygen concentrators deliver oxygen with very little humidity. The most common type of humidification device bubbles oxygen through water to pick up humidity. This device delivers gas that has been humidified to approximately 20% to 30% relative humidity. Use of humidifiers is usually unnecessary when flow rates are exceedingly small.

Oxygen therapy should be monitored in order to maintain adequate oxygen levels and to assess need. The most common monitoring method is to observe the color of the mucous membranes of the mouth and nail beds. Cyanosis, as previously discussed, usually denotes a decreased amount of oxygen in the blood but may be difficult to assess. A more sophisticated method of monitoring oxygen therapy involves the use of pulse oximetry. A pulse oximeter is connected to the patient by means of a clip or taped finger probe. It measures the oxygen content of blood by sensing a change in color between oxygenated and unoxygenated red blood cells. This value is reported as the percentage of blood that is saturated with oxygen, or oxygen saturation. Acceptable values range from about 92% to 99%; lower levels may be acceptable in the child with congenital heart disease. Any cyanotic child or child with a decreased oxygen saturation requires immediate medical attention.

MECHANICAL SUPPORTS

Continuous positive airway pressure

Continuous positive airway pressure (CPAP) is being used more and more frequently as an intermediate step during the process of weaning children from mechanical ventilation. As its name implies, CPAP involves the continuous application of distending pressure to the airway. While CPAP does assist somewhat during inspiration, its chief advantage seems to lie in the maintenance of lung volume during exhalation. It prevents the lungs from completely emptying, thereby preventing collapse of alveoli in diseased lungs. This effect is very similar to the effect of grunting, a maneuver often performed by infants to maintain lung volume (as described in Part I of this series). Even individuals not on ventilatory support experience a level of CPAP, that being the normal atmospheric or barometric pressure. In normal individuals, this level is thought to be somewhere in the range of 2 to 3 cm H_2O. When used as part of an outpatient therapeutic strategy, CPAP in the range of 5 to 10 cm H_2O is typically used.

CPAP can be provided by two different mechanisms. Most CPAP devices for home use generate pressure by producing air flow. The higher the CPAP required, the greater the air flow necessary to maintain that pressure. Some patients, especially younger patients, find the sensation of this air flow extremely uncomfortable and may not tolerate it well. CPAP may also be generated by applying resistance to exhalation. This approach is generally done by using a one-way valve that can be adjusted to provide variable levels of resistance to exhalation. These valves use either a spring or a column of water to provide the resistance to air flow. Most

CPAP devices incorporate an alarm system, alerting caretakers to changes in pressure within the system. This alarm is a very important feature for pediatric patients because they frequently either inadvertently or deliberately remove or dislodge their mask or circuit.

In the home setting CPAP is often delivered by use of a simple mask. This mask may be either a nasal mask, which leaves the patient's mouth free, or a full face mask, which covers both the mouth and nose. While nasal masks are more comfortable for most patients, they may not maintain adequate pressure in patients who do not keep their mouths closed. The full face mask avoids this problem, but some patients find this mask less comfortable, and it increases the risk of aspirating (inhaling) stomach contents in patients prone to vomiting. In patients with a tracheostomy CPAP can be delivered directly to the tracheostomy tube.

A more sophisticated form of CPAP has recently become available. BiPAP® (Respironics, Inc, Murrysville, Pennsylvania) is a flow-type device that is capable of delivering two preset levels of pressure. The device delivers a preset level of pressure during the expiratory phase (expiratory positive airway pressure [EPAP]). When it then senses a drop in pressure within the circuit, indicating the initiation of a breath by the patient, it generates a higher preset pressure level (inspiratory positive airway pressure [IPAP]). This device is extremely helpful in patients who require more support than simple CPAP, but who do not need or do not want more sophisticated mechanical ventilation. In particular, it has been shown to benefit patients with progressive neuromuscular disease.

MECHANICAL VENTILATORS

True mechanical ventilation represents the most aggressive form of ventilatory assistance possible. In general, it should be reserved for patients whose respiratory problems have made it impossible for them to maintain adequate ventilation on their own. Many different ventilators with various features are available both for home and hospital use. In this section only the basic aspects of mechanical ventilators are introduced.

Negative pressure ventilation

The earliest mechanical ventilators to experience widespread use in patients with chronic lung disease were negative pressure ventilators or "iron lungs." These ventilators generate air flow into and out of the lungs by mimicking the function of the diaphragm and accessory respiratory muscles. By decreasing the pressure around the chest, the chest wall itself is drawn outward and air flows into the lungs. The negative pressure is then relieved or reversed, the chest wall falls back to its normal position and air is exhaled from the lungs. These devices are most effective in patients with normal lungs whose respiratory failure is caused by neuromuscular disorders. Still in use today, negative pressure ventilation no longer requires the bulk of an iron lung, but can be delivered through use of a shell, or cuirass, surrounding the chest wall or a jacket that is sealed at the neck, wrist, and waist.

Negative pressure ventilators have the advantage of being relatively simple and noninvasive. Their use is generally limited, however, to patients with normal lungs and respiratory failure due to weakness of the respiratory muscles. Use of these devices is also difficult in patients with deformities of the chest wall. Other disadvantages include the inability to control tidal volume precisely (ie, the amount of air being drawn into the chest with each breath) and limited access to the patient.

Positive pressure ventilation

Pressure-limited ventilators produce air flow into the airways until a preset pressure is reached. At that point, flow is discontinued, and the patient is allowed to exhale. Ventilation is controlled by adjusting the amount of pressure used to force air into the lungs. This type of ventilation is most commonly used in small infants, especially premature infants. Like the negative pressure ventilators, pressure-limited ventilators do not readily allow for precise control of tidal volume. In addition, as the compliance, or distensibility, of the lung changes, tidal volume may change significantly.

Volume-limited ventilators deliver a preset volume of gas (tidal volume) with each breath. This volume will be delivered regardless of changes in the patient's lung compliance. In this way, volume-cycled ventilators deliver a more constant tidal volume than do negative pressure or pressure-cycled ventilators.

Regardless of the type of ventilator being used, the number of breaths to be delivered per minute—or the respiratory rate—is set. The patient may or may not breathe spontaneously and in addition to the breaths delivered by the ventilator may "trigger" the ventilator to give a breath by initiating inspiration. As previously mentioned, volume-cycled ventilators deliver a preset volume of gas with each breath. However, the volume of gas that actually reaches the lungs is less than that set due to leaks within the ventilator circuit, compression of gas within the circuit, and "loss" of gas to the compliance or distensibility of the circuit itself. These losses can generally be calculated and accounted for when setting the tidal volume. Volume ventilators also incorporate a pressure limit as a safety feature to prevent overdistention of the patient's lungs should the compliance of the lungs change. Most ventilators also include a low pressure limit or alarm to alert caretakers of disconnection of the circuit.

Some ventilators incorporate positive end-expiratory pressure (PEEP) either as a function of the ventilator itself, or in the form of an expiratory valve within the ventilator circuit. This feature serves to maintain lung volume, much like the grunting produced by infants. The PEEP is generally set in the range of 5 to 10 cm H_2O in the home setting.

In the acute care setting, mechanical ventilation is generally carried out by use of an endotracheal tube (a tube passed through the mouth or nose, through the vocal cords, and into the trachea). Mechanical ventilation in the home setting is generally delivered either by mask or via tracheostomy. Just as with CPAP and BiPAP®, ventilation may be carried out using a nasal mask or a full face mask. This form of ventilation is typically used in children who do not require mechanical ventilation on a full-time basis (eg, only at night or during naps). Patients who are fully ventilator dependent very often have a tracheostomy. Some patients may have a fenestrated tracheostomy. This form of tracheostomy tube has an opening to allow air to pass through the upper airway as well (Fig 4). To facilitate speech in patients with a tracheostomy, one-way valves are sometimes placed over the tracheostomy tube opening. These valves allow inspiration of gas but close during exhalation, thereby forcing air around the tracheostomy tube and through the vocal cords.

SAFETY CONSIDERATIONS

Patient safety

The ability of a child to tolerate the proposed therapy should be assessed jointly by the physician and the therapist. Obviously, this assessment should occur at the

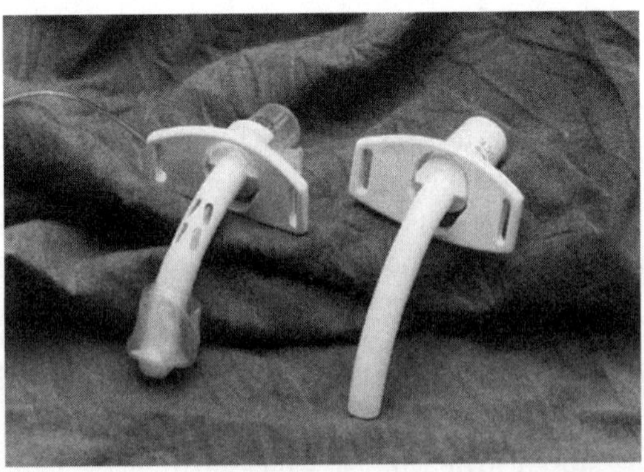

Fig 4. Tracheostomy tubes. Left: a fenestrated, cuffed tracheostomy tube with the cuff deflated. Right: an uncuffed tracheostomy tube.

initial evaluation. Any questions regarding the child's ability to tolerate therapy should be addressed with the patient care team as they arise. Caretakers (patients, nurses, or others) are often a good source of information regarding the tolerance level of a child for particular activities. Some patients may require the presence of a caretaker or other professional staff member (respiratory therapist or nurse). Therapy staff may need special training on relevant equipment to assure patient safety. Likewise, the medical regimen may need to be adjusted before or at the time of therapy (eg, increasing oxygen supplementation, giving an aerosolized medication, or giving chest physiotherapy and suctioning).

Therapeutic sessions should be interrupted or discontinued when any sign of distress occurs. All therapists should be certified in Basic Life Support (BLS) and, if appropriate, certified in Pediatric Advanced Life Support (PALS) as well. Clearly identified contingency plans and lines of communication must be in place (who to notify, when, and how to contact).

Therapist safety

Infants potentially harbor and shed a number of infectious agents that might be harmful to team members. These agents include, but are not limited to, human immunodeficiency virus (HIV); cytomegalovirus (CMV); hepatitis A, B, or C; and a number of respiratory or gastrointestinal viruses (respiratory syncytial virus, influenza, rotovirus). Thus safety considerations dictate the need for strict adherence to universal precautions. Many institutions require yearly training in universal precautions as a prerequisite for continued employment. An institution's infection control committee or the local health department can be valuable sources of information on universal precautions. Questions regarding infection control issues should be addressed with the referring physician and the institutional infection control office.

• • •

Being confronted with a child with respiratory difficulties can be both frightening and intimidating. However, when caregivers understand normal and abnormal lung function and are familiar with the signs and symptoms of significant respiratory distress in infants, they can rapidly identify the children who require evaluation and possible treatment by medical personnel. A number of therapeutic strategies, including interventions designed to normalize pulmonary physiology and mechanical devices to assist pulmonary function, have been presented. Important considerations regarding the safety of both the child and the therapist have also been discussed. It is sincerely hoped that this information will make interdisciplinary caregivers feel more comfortable when working with infants and children with chronic respiratory disorders and enable them to optimize interventions in order to help these children obtain their full potential.

Use of surfactant in premature infants: How it affects health and developmental outcomes

Robert J. Boyle, MD
Associate Professor of Pediatrics
Department of Pediatrics
University of Virginia Health Sciences Center
Charlottesville, Virginia

RESPIRATORY DISTRESS SYNDROME (RDS) represents the most important medical problem of the premature infant. RDS causes the majority of deaths and, together with conditions closely related to it, is responsible for much of the short- and long-term illness associated with preterm birth. Immediately or shortly after birth, infants with RDS have difficulty breathing, rapid respirations, increasing requirement for oxygen, and in some cases complete respiratory failure. Treatment may involve oxygen therapy, continuous positive airway pressure, and in severe cases tracheal intubation and positive-pressure mechanical ventilation.

BACKGROUND

RDS is the result of abnormal surface tension forces in the air sacs (alveoli) and small airways of the lung that cause the lung to be stiff and difficult to inflate. With expiration, the alveoli and small airways have an increased tendency to collapse (atelectasis). The infant must work harder to attempt to inflate the lung. In addition, as the disease progresses blood plasma proteins leak into the alveoli and airways, and blood flow through the lung decreases. The protein deposits observed microscopically led to the former use of the term *hyaline membrane disease* to describe this process. Infants with RDS become progressively sicker over the first 48 to 72 hours of life. The disease then stabilizes, and on approximately the fourth day of life, if the infant survives and the disease course has been uncomplicated, the infant begins to improve.

The more preterm the infant, the greater the likelihood of RDS. Of infants born at 24 to 26 weeks, 60% to 70% develop the disease; only 5% to 10% of those born at 34-35 weeks are affected. This incidence may be altered by a number of factors, including sex, race, maternal disease, prolonged rupture of the fetal membranes, and multiple pregnancy.

RDS and its treatment are responsible for the development of bronchopulmonary dysplasia (BPD), which may require long-term hospitalization, weeks to months of mechanical ventilation, and oxygen therapy. BPD is also associated with a high incidence of developmental delay.[1,2]

RDS is also related directly and indirectly to other conditions that increase the risk of mortality and long-term morbidity for the infant (see the box, "Morbidity Associated with RDS"). Respiratory distress and positive-pressure ventilation in-

Inf Young Children 1993; 6(1): 21–25

crease the risk of lung rupture with air leak into the tissue of the lung (pulmonary interstitial emphysema) and air leak from the lung into the chest cavity (pneumothorax). These are often life-threatening events and increase the risk of intracranial hemorrhage. Sick preterm infants in general have an increased incidence of intraventricular hemorrhage. Severe intraventricular hemorrhage is associated with progressive hydrocephalus and neurodevelopmental abnormality.[3]

Treatment of RDS has evolved over the past 30 to 35 years with the introduction of neonatal intensive care, more sophisticated methods of ventilatory assistance, closely monitored oxygen therapy, and prenatal pharmacologic intervention to delay preterm birth and to accelerate pulmonary maturation. Nevertheless, RDS remains the most important medical hurdle for preterm infants.

SURFACTANT PHYSIOLOGY

Approximately 35 years ago, Pattle[4] discovered an antiatelectasis factor, which lowers the surface tension forces that cause the lung to collapse during expiration. In 1959, Avery and Mead[5] reported that lungs from infants who had died of RDS lack normal surface tension-lowering properties. Surface tension forces make the walls of the alveoli tend to collapse and stick together when the infant exhales. Early investigation showed that this surface tension-lowering factor, or surfactant, contains lecithin. Several clinical trials using instilled or aerosolized lecithin in infants with RDS in the 1960s were unsuccessful.

Since that early experience, a number of investigators continued to investigate surfactant composition, production, biophysics, function, and genetics. It is now recognized that natural surfactant is a complex mixture of lipids and proteins. Sur-

Morbidity Associated with RDS

- Short-term morbidities
  - Pneumothorax
  - Pulmonary interstitial emphysema
  - BPD
  - Intraventricular hemorrhage
  - Posthemorrhagic hydrocephalus
  - Patent ductus arteriosus
  - Necrotizing enterocolitis
  - Apnea of prematurity
- Long-term morbidities
  - Retinopathy of prematurity
  - Hearing loss
  - Developmental delay
  - Cerebral palsy

factant is produced and stored in the cells of the lung beginning at approximately gestation week 24. As gestation progresses, surfactant storage and release increase, so that by 34 to 35 weeks most infants have sufficient surfactant activity. Surfactant functions to keep alveoli open and to reduce the work required to inflate the lung.

DEVELOPMENT OF SURFACTANT REPLACEMENT THERAPY

In the 1970s several independent investigators developed both animal-derived and artificial surfactants. In response to concerns about human infant exposure to large amounts of animal protein, the animal-derived surfactant was extracted to remove all but approximately 1% of the foreign protein. Animal studies confirmed that these surfactants—human, natural (bovine or porcine), and artificial—dramatically improved pulmonary function in animals with RDS.

CLINICAL STUDIES

Clinical studies of surfactant in human newborns followed quickly,[6,7] initially with small pilot studies and later with large, multicenter, randomized studies. Initial studies investigated the response of infants with severe RDS to a single dose of surfactant (rescue) and that of infants administered a single dose immediately after birth (prophylaxis). Current protocols allow a prophylactic dose in infants at highest risk for RDS, multiple rescue doses in those with established RDS, or a prophylactic dose followed by additional rescue doses as necessary.

Clinical studies convincingly show that both prophylactic and rescue therapy significantly improve the pulmonary status of treated infants (see the box, "Results of Surfactant Replacement Therapy"). There are dramatic differences between control and treated infants in peak oxygen requirement, ventilator settings, duration of oxygen therapy, and duration of mechanical ventilation. In addition, most studies have shown a significant decrease in mortality and short-term morbidities.

OTHER RDS-RELATED MORBIDITY

Even with surfactant therapy, there continues to be a significant incidence of moderate and severe RDS, BPD, and death. In addition, few studies have demonstrated a significant reduction in other morbidities associated with prematurity and RDS, including intraventricular hemorrhage, retinopathy of prematurity, sepsis, necrotizing enterocolitis, and prolonged oxygen requirement. In extremely low-birth weight infants (less than 1000 g), surfactant therapy may prevent the acute respiratory distress, but many of these infants develop a chronic oxygen require-

Results of Surfactant Replacement Therapy

Decreased incidence/severity of respiratory distress
- Peak oxygen requirement
- Peak and mean ventilator pressure requirements
- Duration of oxygen therapy
- Duration of mechanical ventilation

Decreased short-term morbidities
- Pneumothorax
- Pulmonary interstitial emphysema
- BPD

Decreased mortality

ment several weeks after birth that may not be related to surfactant status. This highlights the fact that these other clinical problems have multifactorial etiologies.

DEVELOPMENTAL FOLLOW-UP

Although many published studies report improvements in mortality, respiratory severity, and short-term morbidity, there are few published long-term developmental follow-up studies. Vaucher et al[8] assessed postnatal growth and neurodevelopmental outcome in a group of infants enrolled in a controlled rescue trial using human surfactant. There were no significant differences between the treated and control infants with respect to growth and neurologic or developmental outcome as determined by a number of assessment tools. Although not statistically significant, there was a trend toward decreased incidence of spastic cerebral palsy (14% in the treated group compared to 28% in the controls). The incidence of posthemorrhagic hydrocephalus requiring ventriculoperitoneal shunting was similar in both groups (18%).

In a 2-year follow-up study of infants enrolled in a prophylaxis trial with a relatively small sample size, Dunn et al[9] also found no significant differences between treated and control infants in growth and developmental, neurologic, or sensory status. Although more of the control infants died in the neonatal period (2.5% treated compared to 18.2% untreated), 17% of the surviving treated infants compared to 8% of the surviving controls had a major neurodevelopmental handicap (blindness, cerebral palsy leading to functional limitation, and/or Bayley score less than 50). Two of the treated infants were blind secondary to retinopathy of prematurity. The incidence of minor developmental handicap (sensorimotor abnormality not leading to significant functional limitation and/or Bayley score between 50 and 68) was 16% in both groups. Seventy-six percent of the controls and 67% of the treated group were classified as normal.

In a study of extremely high-risk infants weighing 600 to 750 g at birth who were enrolled in a multiple-dose trial of surfactant beginning shortly after birth, Ferrara et al[10] also noted no significant difference in the incidence of mild to moderate abnormality of significant impairment among the survivors followed to 1 year of age. In this study, the treated group had a significantly higher survival rate (81% compared to 50%). Of the total population, 53% of the treated infants survived with a normal outcome compared to 25% of the control infants.

Although there are no published follow-up studies with larger populations, it is evident that a significantly higher percentage of infants treated with surfactant replacement survive their neonatal course. This is especially impressive for infants born weighing less than 1000 g. Although there are more survivors after preterm birth, surfactant therapy does not appear to alter the incidence of abnormal neurodevelopmental outcome for surviving infants. There are only a few published studies, but the incidence of developmental delay, spastic diplegia, and visual impairment secondary to retinopathy of prematurity is similar with or without surfactant therapy. This would suggest that the causes of these long-term morbidities are multifactorial, involving prenatal, medical, and social factors, so that altering the incidence and severity of RDS may have little effect on their incidence.

• • •

Basic research on surfactant biochemistry and physiology has led to the development of multiple natural and artificial surfactants available for replacement therapy for RDS. Both animal and human clinical studies have demonstrated a dramatic effect in preventing RDS and in treating established RDS. Treated infants have significantly lower disease severity, require less support with oxygen and ventilator therapy, experience less BPD, and have significantly higher survival rates. Acute complications due to air leak are reduced.

Nevertheless, RDS-related long-term developmental abnormalities for survivors do not appear to be reduced after otherwise effective surfactant therapy. Larger studies with many more subjects and appropriate consideration of confounding variables will be required to assess the more subtle effects of surfactant on developmental outcomes.

REFERENCES

1. Bregman J, Farrell EE. Neurodevelopmental outcome in infants with bronchopulmonary dysplasia. *Clin Perinatol.* 1992;19:673–694.
2. Bozynski ME. Comprehensive management of the infant with bronchopulmonary dysplasia: a growing challenge. *Infants Young Child.* 1989;2:14–24.
3. Vaucher YE. Understanding intraventricular hemorrhage and white-matter injury in premature infants. *Infants Young Child.* 1988;1:31–45.

4. Pattle KE. Properties, function and origin of the alveolar lining layer. *Nature (London).* 1955;175:1125–1126.
5. Avery ME, Mead J. Surface properties in relation to atelectasis and hyaline membrane disease. *Am J Dis Child.* 1959;97:517–523.
6. Fujiwara T, Chida S, Watabe Y, et al. Artificial surfactant therapy in hyaline membrane disease. *Lancet.* 1980;1:55–59.
7. Smyth JA, Metcalfe IL, Duffy P, et al. Hyaline membrane disease treated with bovine surfactant. *Pediatrics.* 1983;71:913–917.
8. Vaucher YE, Merritt TA, Hallman M, et al. Neurodevelopmental and respiratory outcome in early childhood after human surfactant treatment. *Am J Dis Child.* 1988;142:927–930.
9. Dunn MS, Shennan AT, Hoskins EM, Lennox K, Enhorning G. Two-year follow-up of infants enrolled in a randomized trial of surfactant replacement therapy for prevention of neonatal respiratory distress syndrome. *Pediatrics.* 1988;82:543–547.
10. Ferrara TB, Hoekstra RE, Couser RJ, et al. Effects of surfactant therapy on outcome of infants with birth weights of 600 to 750 grams. *J Pediatr.* 1991;119:455–457.

Index

R

S

T